Community Emergency Medicine

For Elsevier:

Commissioning Editor: Robert Edwards
Development Editor: Catherine Jackson/Rebecca Gleave
Project Manager: Andrew Palfreyman
Designer: Sarah Russell
Illustration Buyer: Gillian Richards
Illustrator: Tim Loughhead

Community Emergency Medicine

Edited by

Jim Wardrope MBChB FRCS FCEM

Consultant in Emergency Medicine,
Northern General Hospital, Sheffield, UK

Peter Driscoll MBChB BSc MD FRCS FCEM

Consultant in Emergency Medicine, Hope Hospital, Salford, UK

Colville Laird MBChB DRCOG FIMS RCS(Ed)

Director of Education, Basics Education Scotland, Scotland, UK

Malcolm Woollard MPH MBA MA(Ed) DipIMC(RCSEd) PGCE RN SRPara FASI

Consultant Paramedic and Director, Faculty of Pre-Hospital Care Research Unit, Visiting
Professor in Pre-hospital Emergency Care, University of Teeside, Teeside, UK

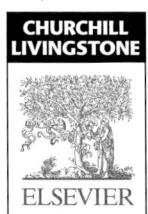

CHURCHILL
LIVINGSTONE

ELSEVIER

EDINBURGH   LONDON   NEW YORK   OXFORD   PHILADELPHIA   ST LOUIS   SYDNEY   TORONTO   2008

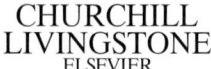

CHURCHILL
LIVINGSTONE
ELSEVIER

First published 2008

ISBN 1: 978-0-443-10325-4

British Library Cataloguing in Publication Data
A catalogue record for this book is available from the British Library

Library of Congress Cataloging in Publication Data
A catalog record for this book is available from the Library of Congress

Note
Knowledge and best practice in this field are constantly changing. As new research and experience broaden our knowledge, changes in practice, treatment and drug therapy may become necessary or appropriate. Readers are advised to check the most current information provided (i) on procedures featured or (ii) by the manufacturer of each product to be administered, to verify the recommended dose or formula, the method and duration of administration, and contraindications. It is the responsibility of the practitioner, relying on their own experience and knowledge of the patient, to make diagnoses, to determine dosages and the best treatment for each individual patient, and to take all appropriate safety precautions. To the fullest extent of the law, neither the publisher nor the editors assumes any liability for any injury and/or damage.

The Publisher

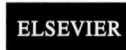

your source for books,
journals and multimedia
in the health sciences

www.elsevierhealth.com
Printed in China

The
Publisher's
policy is to use
**paper manufactured
from sustainable forests**

Contents

Contributors

Elizabeth Jane Blowers RGN RMN BSc(Hons) PGDip
Mental Health Lecturer, University of East Anglia, Norwich, UK

Derek Burroughs
Lecturer, Mental Health and Learning Disability, University of East Anglia, Norwich, UK

Sarah Carter MBChB MRCGP DRCOG
General Practitioner, BASICS Education Scotland, Auchterarder, UK

Rosie Doy
Deputy Director of Teaching and Learning, University of East Anglia, Norwich, UK

Peter Driscoll MBChB BSc MD FRCS FCEM
Consultant in Emergency Medicine, Hope Hospital, Salford, UK

Chris Fitzsimmons MBChB, FCEM
Consultant in Emergency Medicine, Sheffield Children's Hospital, Sheffield, UK

Diana Jane Fothergill MBChB FRCOG
Consultant Obstetrician and Gynaecologist, Sheffield Teaching Hospitals, Sheffield, UK

Carole Gavin (previously Libetta) MRCP FRCS(Ed) FCEM MD
Consultant in Emergency Medicine, Hope Hospital, Salford, UK

James Gray MBChB MRCS DipPHIC MRCGP
General Practitioner, Community Medical Advisor, Yorkshire Ambulance Service, Sheffield, UK

Ian Greaves MBChB FRCP FCEM FIMC RCSEd DTMeH DipMedEd
Professor of Emergency Medicine, The James Cook University Hospital, Middlesbrough, UK

John Hall MBChB DRCOG Dip IMC RCS(Ed)
General Practitioner and Hon. Lecturer in Emergency Care, University of Birmingham, Birmingham, UK

Fiona Jewkes MBChB FRCPCH
General Practitioner, Paediatrician, Medical Director of Wiltshire Ambulance Service, UK

Colville Laird MBChB DRCOG FIMS RCS(Ed)
Director of Education, BASICS Education Scotland, Scotland, UK

Mike Langran MBChB MRCGP
General Practitioner, Aviemore Health Centre, Scotland, UK

Peter Lawson MBChB FRCP
Consultant Physician and Geriatrician, Sheffield Teaching Hospitals, Sheffield, UK

Roderick MacKenzie MBChB FCEM
Consultant in Emergency Medicine, Director of MAGPAS, St Ives Cambridge, UK

Chris Richmond
Emergency Care Practitioner, Yorkshire Ambulance Service, Rotherham, UK

John Scott MBChB
Medical Director, East of England Ambulance Trust, UK

Emma Sutton RMN BSc(Hons) PGDip MA
Lecturer, Nursing and Midwifery, University of East Anglia, Norwich, UK

Jim Wardrope MBChB FRCS FCEM
Consultant in Emergency Medicine, Northern General Hospital, Sheffield, UK

Malcolm Woollard MPH MBA MA(Ed) DipIMC(RCSEd) PGCE RN SRPara FASI
Consultant Paramedic and Director, Faculty of Pre-Hospital Care Research Unit, Visiting Professor in Pre-hospital Emergency Care, University of Teeside, Teeside, UK

Preface

The demand for emergency care has never been higher. New ways of working are required to meet the needs of patients in the community and to reduce the reliance on secondary care. A number of new roles have been created in this environment but there is a lack of the academic literature to support these new roles.

Community Emergency Medicine sets out to describe a system of making a swift assessment of a patient to identify the few who will need immediate life-saving treatment and those who will need to go to hospital. This is based on the system of 'primary survey' that will be familiar to all those with training in the care of the acutely ill patient. These patients will require rapid transport to hospital, often with treatment during the journey.

However, a large majority of patients will not have an immediately life-threatening problem and the text uses a system that will be familiar to many in primary care, 'SOAP-C', to provide a framework for the history taking (Subjective information), examination/tests (Objective information), Analysis of the problem leading to a Plan of management. We have added Communication with other parts of the health and social care system, and with patients and carers – a vital part of an increasingly complex emergency care system.

More patient care is being delivered along pathways of care. These will vary between different health communities. This book tries to take variations in practice into account but each practitioner will need to be aware of local policy regarding the details of each care and referral pathway.

Emergency care is never easy, but the use of a system to guide assessment and care has been very successful in the care of patients requiring resuscitation. The authors and editors hope that a simple system to aid the assessment and care of less acute, but more common problems. It should assist doctors in emergency primary care and emergency medicine, emergency care practitioners, minor illness practitioners, first contact practitioners, advanced paramedics – those at the 'sharp end' of medical care.

Jim Wardrope
Sheffield 2007

Acknowledgements

This book is based on the series 'The ABC of Community Emergency Medicine' that appeared in the Emergency Medicine Journal 2004–2005. We would like to thank BMJ publications for their support and help in the writing of the series and allowing us to use that material for this book. We would like to thank all those who have contributed to the project. We thank the publishing team at Elsevier for their support and encouragement.

The system of 'primary survey/secondary survey' is taken from life support courses, especially the Advanced Trauma Life Support Course. The SOAP system is taken from works on the problem-orientated method.

The Medical Illustration Department, Northern General Hospital, Sheffield provided the photographs and illustrations in Chapters 2 and 13. Fiona Mair of BASICS Education Scotland and Sue Wieteska of the Advanced Life Support Group provided the photographs used in Chapters 4 and 5.

We would like to dedicate the book to those involved in making the difficult decisions in emergency care. We hope that general practitioners, paramedics, ECPs, minor illness practitioners and first contact practitioners will find the book helpful.

We also thank our long-suffering wives and families for their patience and support during the production of this book.

Jim Wardrope, Colville Laird and Peter Driscoll

Introduction, summary, the system of care

Introduction

In the UK and in other countries there is a growing shortage of trained clinicians to meet the need for immediate assessment and treatment of urgent medical problems in primary care. Traditionally doctors have been the main providers of this care but already nurses, paramedics, and other healthcare professionals are extending their role to include clinical assessment, decision making, and treatment.[1,2] Our aim is that this book will be a useful update for general practitioners experienced in this field and also serve as an introduction to those new to emergency clinical decision making.

We will describe the management of non-traumatic emergencies commonly encountered in community emergency care. The objective is to provide a clear and easily followed system of assessment and management of the ill patient.

This system will teach a method for the rapid recognition and treatment of immediately life threatening problems or conditions that require urgent hospital care. However, the focus of the book is the assessment of patients with less serious problems who can be managed without referral to hospital.

The book will use *presentations* rather than diagnoses as the starting point, for example the approach to the breathless patient rather than the treatment of asthma; the care of the disturbed patient rather than the diagnosis of specific mental illness.

Where possible we will try to make recommendations based on evidence. The field of emergency medicine is not rich in scientific analysis and community emergency care even less. We will interpret and transfer as much of the evidence as possible into the community emergency care setting.

Lastly and perhaps most importantly, the book sets the immediate management in the context of the start of the patient's journey. The key principle (Box 1.1) is – *what is right for this patient, in this setting, with my skills, at this time?* There is evidence that some pre-hospital interventions may make patient outcomes worse. Just because a particular line of management *can* be practiced out of hospital it does not necessarily mean that it *should* be done.

BOX 1.1 **Key points**

- Immediate treatment is often only the first part of the patient's care. The immediate management must be seen as part of the continuum of care.
- Just because an intervention *can* be carried out does not mean that it is always in the patient's best interests to do so.

> **BOX 1.2 Book outline**
>
> - Introduction
> - The system of assessment and the resuscitation of the primary survey positive patient
> - Airway and breathing problems
> - Chest pain
> - Neurological abnormalities and poisoning
> - ENT/dermatological conditions
> - Falls and the elderly population
> - Gynaecology and obstetrics/abdominal pain
> - The acutely disturbed patient/mental health
> - Fever/nausea and vomiting in the unwell adult
> - The assessment of the unwell child
> - Paediatric presentations
> - Musculoskeletal problems
> - Systems design, communications, ethics

Scope

The book outline is given in Box 1.2. This encompasses most of acute emergency medicine. Trauma is occasionally mentioned as it can be part of the presenting complaint (for example, in a collapse with an injury) or a possible cause (for example, in chest pain). However we will not deal with serious trauma as this is well covered in other texts.

Chapter format

The chapters will start with a list of objectives then go on to discuss the care of the 'primary survey positive' patient, identify the types of serious problems requiring hospital admission, and concentrate on describing the assessment and management of patients who might be treated at home.

The three step system of care

Overview

We will use a *three step system of care* (Box 1.3). The first step is to identify those patients with immediately life threatening problems, the second is to identify those patients who will need to go to hospital, and the third to fully assess that majority of patients encountered in community emergency care that will not require hospital referral. There may be no single 'right answer' to the immediate management of each of these problems. The variables in levels of training,

BOX 1.3 **The system of care**

Figures from out-of-hours contacts to primary care in the UK indicate that only 1–2% of patients will require resuscitation. Most patients will have conditions that can be managed at home.
- Step 1 – identify those patients with immediately life threatening problems, provide essential initial resuscitation and transport
- Step 2 – identify those patients with conditions requiring immediate hospital care, provide essential treatment and transport
- Step 3 – fully assess all other patients and decide on the appropriate management of the patient

distance or time to definitive care will influence the decision on the right management for this patient at this time and in this place (see below).

We will designate a patient as *primary survey positive* if a potentially life threatening problem is identified. In such cases the two major objectives are to administer those treatments or interventions that are absolutely essential and to prepare the patient for transport.

Step 1

The first step is to identify those patients who are 'primary survey positive'. This process will usually take less than 30 seconds. If the patient is talking in full sentences, is fully orientated, the respiratory rate is between 10 and 29 breaths per minute, the pulse rate between 50 and 120, and the patient is not cold and sweating, then it is unlikely they need immediate resuscitation (Box 1.4).

Step 2

The next step is to identify the patient who obviously needs hospital admission, especially if the treatment needs to be given as soon as possible to reduce risk to life or limb (Box 1.5). Examples would be acute myocardial infarction, bleeding, suspected aortic aneurysm or imminent

BOX 1.4 **Quick assessment of the primary survey in adults**

Patients fulfilling all these criteria are unlikely to have an immediately life threatening problem:
- can talk in complete sentences
- fully alert
- respiratory rate is between 10 and 29 breaths per minute
- pulse is between 50 and 120 beats per minute
- patient is not cold, clammy, or sweaty

BOX 1.5 **Criteria that identify patients requiring immediate life saving intervention**

- A: potential airway compromise
  - unconscious patient/stridor/anaphylaxis/Hx of FB
- B: severe respiratory distress
  - respiratory rate >10 or greater than 29 (adult)
  - O_2 sats <93% on air
- C: clinical signs of shock
  - pulse <50 or >120 (adult)
  - systolic BP < 90 mmHg
- D: GCS less 12 (acute deterioration)
  - (acute stroke)
- Obstetric emergency (not routine childbirth)

childbirth. In these patients essential treatment should be provided and transport to the appropriate hospital arranged.

Step 3

Most patients will need a full assessment to reach a decision about treatment and ongoing care. A system to aid this assessment is outlined later in this chapter. The overall approach to community emergency care is illustrated as a decision tree in Figure 1.1.

Fig. 1.1 Decision tree for the system of care.

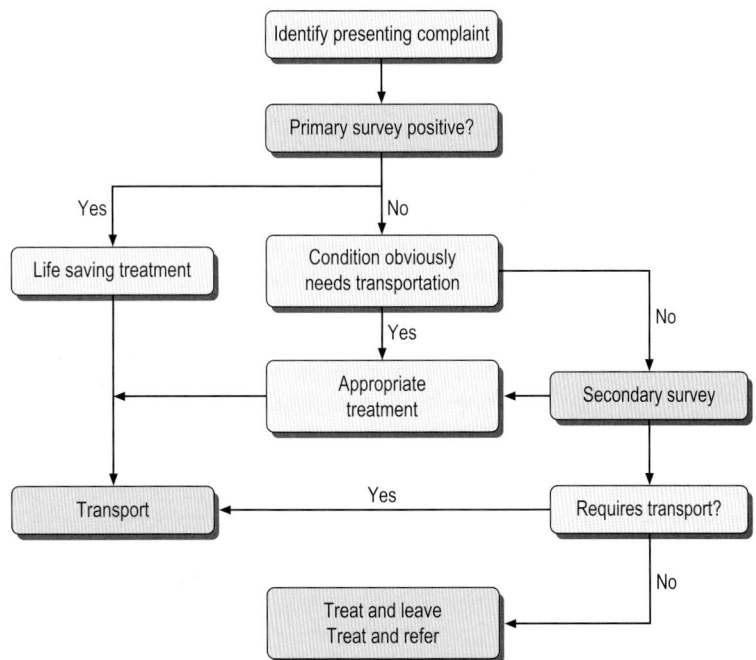

Primary survey positive

Which treatment does the patient need now?

There are some conditions that demand immediate treatment. For example, the outcomes of cardiac arrest are dependent on the time to defibrillation; anaphylaxis needs epinephrine, and an obstructed airway requires urgent attention. However, in many other conditions the evidence is not so clear. The principle should be to do the minimum necessary while preparing for transport and to continue treatment en route. Life threatening asthma would be a good example. Starting an oxygen-driven salbutamol nebuliser and ensuring there were no signs of a tension pneumothorax would be the main on scene interventions. Rapid transport to hospital would be the next priority with en route treatment and evaluation as necessary.

 TIP

Primary survey positive: action – arrange transport and provide essential treatment

Do I need to transport immediately?

For most patients with a critical illness the best treatment is transfer to a facility capable of critical care. It can be tempting to try to 'stabilise the patient' but vital minutes can be lost. The patient with the life threatening asthma needs to be in an environment where emergent ventilation and cardiovascular support can be provided safely and quickly.

Do I need back up?

If the patient has a critical problem there will be very few situations where you will require back up to travel to you. The time involved in mobilising such assistance may outweigh any treatment gains.

Patient obviously requires hospital treatment

Many patients will have conditions requiring hospital care. Box 1.6 lists some that need emergency transfer. However, the patient with a fracture neck of femur requires a brief history, vital signs, pain relief and written notes including a treatment plan. This allows their care in hospital to be a continuum rather than simply repetition of the pre-hospital assessment.

BOX 1.6 Emergency transfer

Any of these criteria would mark the patient as requiring immediate transfer to hospital:
- suspected acute MI
- suspected acute blood loss (for example, GI or aortic aneurysm)
- suspected acute vascular occlusion

Secondary survey

Patient stable, no immediate reason for hospital transport

The decision to assess, treat, and leave requires much more care and judgement than the decision to transfer to hospital. It also carries higher risk. Equally the whole system would be swamped if all patients were sent to hospital. In some presenting complaints, for example chest pain, a high proportion of patients will require hospital evaluation. Other complaints such as a sore throat will rarely need anything other than advice or simple treatment. To minimise the risk it is essential that clinicians carry out a systematic assessment. We outline one such system – SOAPC[3] (Box 1.7). There are many others. It is not important which you use, as long as you use a system that includes all the key elements.

BOX 1.7 Secondary survey, treatment, and ongoing care

- Subjective information – presenting complaint(s), history of complaint(s), previous history, social information
- Objective information – general exam, targeted specific exam, other exam, tests, vital signs
- Analysis – differential diagnosis: most likely, most serious, common pitfalls
- Plan – treat and transport, treat and refer, treat and leave
- Communication – patient explanation/understanding/questions/choice/safety netting/receiving unit/responsible adult carer

---

Subjective information gathering: the history

Where there is a definite pathology, a full understanding of the history of the patient's problem will give very clear pointers to the diagnosis in the majority of cases.[4] Examination and tests may help confirm the provisional diagnosis but the history remains the key tool of the emergency care clinician.

The process of history taking can be conveniently broken down into the components shown in Box 1.8. Elicit and record the patient's chief complaint. This will often direct the clinician down a particular line of thought or specific care pathway. However, always be willing to change direction as other evidence is obtained. It is very common for presenting complaints to change over time as a disease develops. The initial symptoms of influenza, meningitis and pneumonia may be identical, making the diagnosis difficult or impossible. Within 6 hours the patient may have developed the rash, photophobia and neck stiffness or the

> ### BOX 1.8 Key parts of the history
>
> - Presenting complaint(s), symptom onset, progress of symptoms, associated symptoms, previous treatment for this episode
> - Previous history of similar symptoms
> - Other medical history
> - Drugs/allergies
> - Social history/circumstances/tobacco–alcohol–drugs

pleuritic chest pain, breathlessness and green sputum that would allow a layman to make the diagnosis. The initial consultation assesses the patient at one point in the disease process, the emergency care clinician can return to re-assess the patient's progress.

The detailed inquiry into the onset and progress of these symptoms often gives a clear mental picture of the patient's problem. Associated symptoms also need to be recorded and, in some conditions, a targeted systematic inquiry is carried out. For example, in the patient with pleuritic chest pain you should ask about shortness of breath/sputum/haemoptysis/leg pain.

This may not be the first time the patient has sought advice for this problem. This can be a danger in healthcare systems that are becoming increasingly complex with many access points to care. Beware of simply confirming a diagnosis given by another health professional. Be extra vigilant if this is the third call for help for the same problem.

Medical history, current medications, and allergies should be recorded. This is made easy by using a proforma history sheet (see later).

Social history is an ever increasing factor in the assessment of the emergency care needs of patients. The frail elderly living at the margins of safety often have greater social care requirements than medical needs.

A final word of warning, if there are problems in obtaining a clear history take extra care in your assessment and treatment planning. This is such a vital part of the decision making process that without a clear history the confidence of any particular diagnosis will be greatly reduced. The very young, the very old, those with language problems or learning difficulties are some of the situations where the lack of history causes clear problems.

TIP

The holistic care of the emergency patient is the hallmark of an integrated emergency care system.

PITFALL

Lack of history increases assessment problems in:
- Babies and infants
- The older patient
- Patients with learning problems
- Patients whose first language is not English

Objective information gathering

Examination

Vital signs (temperature, pulse, blood pressure, respiratory rate and oxygen saturation) are often the first and most important indicator of the severity of a patient's illness. They provide an objective measure of the patient's physiology at the time of the examination. As noted in Box 1.3 vital signs are key in spotting those patients who are primary survey positive. Vital signs may be normal in many life threatening situations (acute MI is the obvious example) – a patient's condition can change rapidly. Fail to record vital signs, or to take heed of abnormal readings, at your peril.

General examination focuses on the systemic signs of disease. Identifying the unwell patient is one of the key skills for any emergency clinician. It is hard to describe the grey, anxious, and slightly dehydrated appearance of the patient with serious illness but clues are to be observed in the general demeanour, the face and eyes, the tongue, skin colour, and turgor (Box 1.9).

BOX 1.9 System of examination

- Vital signs – pulse, blood pressure, respiratory rate oxygen saturation, temperature, GCS, (AMTS)
- General – Is the patient unwell? – colour, rash, sweaty, hydration, eyes, mouth
- Complaint specific – careful examination of the system(s) involved
- Associated systems – other examinations, perhaps remote from site of the presenting complaint
- Other systems – general screening

Complaint specific examination concentrates on the system(s) indicated by the history. There are many books on physical examination and Chapter 2 provides a reasonable standard for community emergency care. Develop a system of examination such as 'look, feel, listen' or 'look, feel, move' appropriate to the part of the body being examined.

Associated systems may need to be examined as part of the routine in specific complaints. Consequently an elderly patient with back pain should have their abdomen examined, their peripheral pulses checked, and a neurological examination of the legs.

It is impossible to perform a full detailed physical examination of every system in the patient's home.

Tests

There are few investigations currently available in the community emergency care setting. The most common are listed in Box 1.10. The 12-lead electrocardiograph (ECG) is perhaps the most useful. Do not place too

> **BOX 1.10 Common community emergency care investigations**
>
> - Electrocardiograph
> - Peak expiratory flow rate (PEFR)
> - Blood glucose
> - Urine

much reliance on a single test. For example, in acute chest pain the initial ECG will be normal in 50% of patients who are having an acute myocardial infarct.[5] If someone has a very typical history of ischaemic chest pain then there is a very high *clinical suspicion* (high pre-test probability) of ischaemic heart disease. In such cases a normal ECG would not influence the referral to hospital. Investigations are probably more important in patients who are going to be left at home. The types and scope of such investigations is likely to increase in the future.

Analysis – differential diagnosis

Use the information gathered in the history and examination to assess the likely cause of the patient's problem. It may not be possible to reach a definite 'diagnosis' but this is not important if the patient is being referred to hospital. In contrast, where the patient is being left at home, a working diagnosis is essential. There is often a degree of uncertainty around any initial diagnosis so try to keep an open mind on alternatives. For example, the patient with sudden onset of severe headache will most likely have a migraine or a tension headache but they might have a subarachnoid haemorrhage. In the series we will try to list the most common diagnoses for each presentation along with some of the 'red flags' (example below) where it is recognised that a serious diagnosis is often overlooked.

RED FLAG

The early signs and symptoms of meningococcal septicaemia are identical to those of influenza

Plan – treatment and ongoing care

Treat and transport

Patients requiring a journey to hospital for further investigation or treatment need an explanation, necessary pre-hospital treatment, and preparation for transfer. Ensure that the notes are completed including a suggested further treatment plan. Local guidelines should enable you to refer the patient to the appropriate department.

Treat and refer

Such patients have a problem that does not need hospital treatment but do require further assessment or treatment. Common examples are the older patient with social care needs or patients requiring community nursing support. Each health system will need to develop a range of clearly defined pathways for referral. Again documentation and a clear treatment plan are essential.

Treat and leave

Many patients will not require transport or referral. These patients will have minor self limiting illnesses or illnesses that can be easily treated at home. The patient should feel that they can seek further advice and assessment if the condition does not improve.

Communication – patient and carer

In all encounters in emergency care there is a duty to communicate effectively with the patient. The patient should understand the treatment plans and be given an opportunity to ask questions. It is good practice to confirm that the patient and carers agree with the plan but it may not be possible to comply with all their wishes. Most health systems have constraints on what can be provided. Alternatives might be to refer the patient to the primary care team for further evaluation.

Communication and records

Keeping good records is one of the key duties of healthcare professionals. In the past records have often been minimalist. In the UK there is a move to electronic patient records but it is likely that paper records will be the norm in many areas for the foreseeable future. The use of semi-proforma records may help the recording of assessments, treatments, and care plans.

 TIP

Patients should feel confident that if their condition deteriorates or does not improve as predicted they can seek further help, preferably from the same service

The variables in community emergency care

The patient

From the newborn child to the 100-year-old woman, from the fit young man having a cardiac arrest playing sport to the dangerously overweight patient on multiple medications, the community emergency care practitioner has to deal with all situations as they present. There is no immediate access to paediatricians, surgeons or the intensive care specialist. The community emergency care practitioner has only their own skills and judgement and training. Increasingly they may be able to use telemedicine or even the humble telephone for a second opinion but they are the clinicians on the spot. Judgement is required to consider how an individual with all their previous history and current circumstances will fit into a specific care pathway (Box 1.11).

BOX 1.11 Variables to consider in deciding on plan of care

- Patient age
- Patient social circumstances
- Patient co-existing disease
- Clinician training and empowerment
- Distance and time to definitive care

The disease (or co-existing diseases)

Airline pilots have it easy. They deal with systems that are mostly predictable, well maintained, and have time and assistance to carry out cross checks. However even with the benefit of these systems they can still make significant errors. Patients are heterogeneous, the response to disease is hugely variable and co-existing diseases modify presentation or treatment. In community emergency care there cannot be cross checks on every action and decision.

The level of competency/the level of empowerment

The old demarcations between healthcare professionals are disappearing and are likely to disappear as new ways of delivering health care become established. However, for the foreseeable future emergency care will be delivered by healthcare professionals with different levels of training and working to different levels of empowerment. The treatment of an acute myocardial infarction epitomises this diversity. A paramedic trained in thrombolysis will be competent to deliver this therapy in the patient's home but an urban general practitioner, who has not obtained such training or experience, will not be able to do so. The management of some conditions and their treatment will vary depending on the training/skills/empowerment of the individual practitioner.

The emergency care system, the environment, distance to definitive care

As if the decisions in emergency medicine were not complicated enough, the effects on patient management because of the environment and transport availability and transit time add further difficulties. The priorities in managing a patient with an acute MI in the middle of a snowstorm on the Cairngorm Plateau will be very different to those if that patient were at home, 5 minutes from a major A&E department.

Summary

Community emergency care represents a highly complex situation in which a very wide variety of conditions are managed by different types of practitioners with a range of competences. A systematic approach to assessment and management is therefore essential to ensure patients are receiving the correct care, in the correct place, at the correct time. This book describes one such systematic approach.

References

1   Mason S, Wardrope J, Perrin J 2003 Developing the community paramedic practitioner intermediate care support scheme for older people with minor conditions. Emerg Med J 20:196–198
2   Pedley D, Bisset K, Connolly E M et al 2003 Prospective observational study of time saved by pre hospital thrombolysis for ST elevation myocardial infarction delivered by paramedics. BMJ 327:22–26
3   Palmer K T 1998 Notes for the MRCGP, 3rd edn. Blackwell Science, Oxford
4   Hampton J R, Harrison M J B, Mitchell J R A 1975 Relative contributions of history taking, physical examination, and laboratory investigations for diagnosis and management of medical outpatients. BMJ 2:486–489
5   Morris F, Brody W J 2002 ABC of clinical electrocardiography. Acute myocardial infarction. BMJ 324:831–834

CHAPTER

2

Jim Wardrope and Roderick MacKenzie

The system of assessment and care of the primary survey positive patient

Introduction

Emergency situations cause stress, especially if they are unfamiliar or present new and different challenges. Specific life threatening medical emergencies may only be experienced by most practitioners a few times in their career[1,2] and even experienced clinicians require training and practice to maintain confidence and skills. Using a system of care and assessment will improve consistency. This chapter aims to set out a system of assessment for the patient with emergency care needs. It can only offer a framework; proper application will require training, flexibility, common sense, and experience (Box 2.1).

> **BOX 2.1 Objectives**
>
> - To describe a system to identify immediately life threatening problems (the primary survey positive patient)
> - To provide guidance on the management of the primary survey positive patient
> - To introduce the SOAPC system for the full evaluation of a patient who might be suitable to treat and refer or treat and leave

Recognition of immediately life threatening problems

Most patients do not have an immediately life-threatening airway, breathing, circulation, or neurological problem. The patient who is talking normally, is fully orientated, is not pale or sweaty, has no dyspnoea, has a normal pulse, and is not breathless is unlikely to be in immediate danger. However the patient's condition may change very quickly and some need careful monitoring and re-evaluation (for example, the patient with chest pain may have a sudden cardiac arrest). Making decisions about the presence or absence of an immediate threat to life can be difficult. There is evidence that important clinical signs of urgent airway, breathing, circulation, or neurological problems may be easily missed, misinterpreted, or mismanaged in the emergency setting in hospital practice;[1,2] the risk of clinical errors in pre-hospital practice is likely to be greater.

Fortunately, there are common presentations for most acute medical emergencies that can be anticipated. These include shortness of breath, chest pain, abdominal pain, collapse, coma, and seizures (Box 2.2).

> **BOX 2.2 Common emergency presentations**
>
> - Coma
> - Difficulty in breathing
> - Chest pain
> - Collapse with hypotension
> - Collapse with altered consciousness
> - Gastrointestinal bleeding
> - Abdominal pain
> - Headache
> - Seizures

The primary survey positive patient

A number of excellent reference texts and resources exist describing the priorities and immediate actions for assessing acutely unwell patients in the hospital and general practice setting.[3–10] The approach and techniques advocated are equally applicable in the resource limited community care environment and during transport to hospital. Similarly, the ABCDE approach taught on standard life support courses is as applicable to acute medical emergencies as it is to resuscitation from cardiac arrest and the management of major trauma. This structured approach is illustrated in Figure 2.1. This reflects the central doctrine of emergency care that immediate assessment and management of a life threatening condition does not require a precise diagnosis. It also illustrates the importance of considering early transport to definitive care with emergency treatment compared with resuscitation en route.

After ensuring the scene is safe, the practitioner should aim to undertake a rapid primary survey (Box 2.3). In many patients, the primary survey may be completed very quickly. The common pathways to cardiac arrest in acute medical emergencies are airway obstruction, respiratory failure, circulatory failure, and neurological failure. The aim of the primary survey is to seek out evidence of these in order to target specific resuscitative interventions.

If the patient is not talking normally then a more detailed airway assessment is required. Look for signs of obstruction and check that the patient is maintaining and protecting the airway. The unconscious patient is at significant risk of *passive regurgitation* and pulmonary aspiration even if the airway is maintained with simple techniques and positioning. Failure to clear blood, saliva or mucus from the oropharynx and absence of spontaneous swallowing indicate a failure of airway protection. Although the full range of basic and advanced airway

Fig. 2.1 Structured approach to identifying the primary survey positive patient.

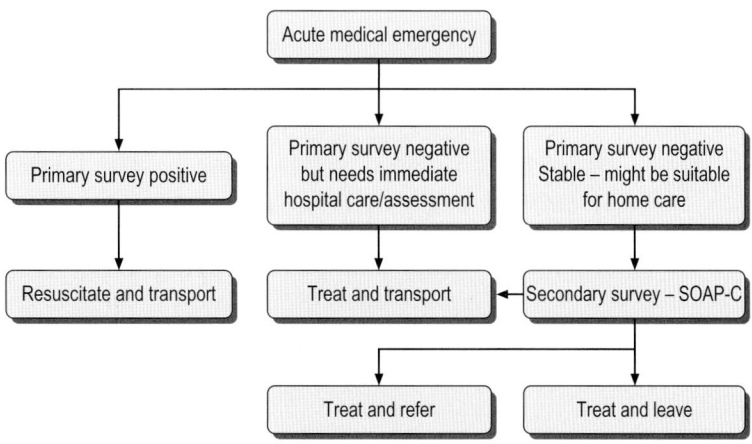

BOX 2.3 Rapid primary survey

Airway Assessment
There is unlikely to be an immediately life threatening airway problem if:
- the patient is talking normally and
- there is no history of anaphylaxis or other airway problems

Breathing Assessment
There is unlikely to be a life threatening breathing problem if:
- the patient is not dyspnoeic
- the respiratory rate is less than 29 and greater than 10 breaths per minute

Circulation Assessment
There is unlikely to be an immediately life threatening circulation problem if:
- the patient's skin is not cold, clammy, sweaty
- the pulse rate is >60 and <120 beats per minute
- there is no evidence of a condition that might cause blood loss
- there are no signs of sepsis
- there is no clinical suspicion that the patient is having an acute myocardial infarct

Disability Assessment
There is unlikely to be an immediately life threatening neurological problem if:
- the patient is fully alert and orientated
- there are no localising neurological deficits (face or limbs)
- there is n o history to suggest meningitis.

The patient's condition can change and this assessment is a continuous process throughout the episode of care

management interventions should be available to manage such patients, simple adjuncts (especially nasopharyngeal airways), postural drainage, and head and neck positioning may be sufficient during the remainder of the primary survey and transfer to hospital.

To assess breathing, look for signs of increased respiratory effort, inadequate ventilation, and common physical signs associated with respiratory and cardiovascular disease. An increased respiratory rate, use of accessory muscles, splinting of the diaphragm, and recession of the chest wall are sensitive indicators of an increased work of breathing. Tachypnoea alone may reflect a very wide range of disease processes and it should not be assumed to reflect a breathing problem in the absence of other signs of respiratory distress. If wheeze is present, decide if the sound occurs mainly during inspiration (*stridor*) or expiration (most likely to be attributable to lower airways obstruction).

Detailed assessment of the circulation should identify the presence of shock and a systemic inflammatory response to infection. Shock is a failure of tissue oxygenation. The classic signs include prolonged capillary refill, tachycardia, tachypnoea, and sympathetic nervous system stimulation (pallor, sweating and peripheral vasoconstriction). 'Sepsis' refers to evidence of systemic infection (for example, pneumonia, meningococcal disease) accompanied by systemic inflammatory responses. These include a pulse rate greater than 90, a respiratory rate greater than 20, and a temperature above 38 °C or below 36 °C. Acute gastrointestinal haemorrhage may be missed if the clinical signs of bleeding are not assessed. Finally, assessment of the circulation in medical emergencies includes an assessment of heart rhythm and a search for evidence of heart failure and myocardial dysfunction (tachycardia, 3rd or 4th heart sounds, systolic murmur).

Detailed assessment of disability entails a mini-neurological examination starting with level of consciousness, mental state, pupil signs, localising signs, posture, and limb function (see below). The patient should also be exposed as much as practicable to look for evidence of a rash (urticaria or purpura), jaundice, anaemia, pitting oedema, and physical manifestations of chronic disease. An accurate assessment of temperature is essential in assessing whether the patient is feverish or hypothermic.

Resuscitation

Resuscitation entails physical interventions and the use of equipment and drugs. The treatment of life threatening airway, breathing, circulation, and neurological problems should take place in parallel with the primary survey.

The range of equipment and drugs available to the practitioner will clearly influence how much can be done. In many cases, simple measures to support the airway, breathing, and circulation while en route to the emergency department are sufficient. There are however conditions where immediate on-scene treatment is essential if life is to be saved. Patients with anaphylaxis, inhaled foreign body, cardiac arrest, myocardial infarction, asthma, continuous seizures, and sepsis for example will usually benefit from immediate intervention at the scene if appropriate equipment and drugs are available. The specific resuscitative interventions for common presentations are discussed in later chapters.

> **TIP**
>
> Start treatment of immediately life threatening problems as they are identified

Patients with a serious illness requiring immediate transport to hospital

There are a number of common problems where the primary survey may confirm that the patient is 'stable' but they may still have a condition that needs immediate treatment, usually in hospital. Chest pain, vascular occlusions, severe shortness of breath, severe abdominal pain, and acute neurological deficit are examples. In such cases the focus of treatment is rapid transport to hospital with any necessary interventions being provided during the journey.

These patients are usually identified during the primary survey and often require little further examination. It is only once life threatening problems have been excluded or identified and treated that a conventional history and examination can be conducted.

The secondary survey

All acutely unwell patients should undergo a primary survey to identify their immediate resuscitation needs but most patients asking for assessment through their primary care service are not likely to need immediate life saving treatment or to be rushed to hospital. There is time to perform a more detailed secondary survey. This follows the more traditional medical model of history and examination.

Any further clinical examination should then be dictated by history and clinical suspicion. A differential diagnosis can then be reached and further decisions made regarding treatment, transportation and definitive care.

TIP

Most patients calling for assessment by their primary care system will not have a serious life threatening problem

The SOAPC system

The system that we have adopted (Box 2.4) is based heavily on problem oriented methodology:[11]

- Subjective information: the history from the patient or carers
- Objective information: examination findings, augmented when appropriate, by investigations and information from the patient record (for example, electronic record or patient held records)
- Analysis: your opinion as to the probable cause of the problem and whether other serious problems need to be ruled out
- Plan: the further care of the patient including advice, treatment with drugs, whether the patient requires another healthcare facility or can stay at home with appropriate follow up and 'safety net' advice
- Communication with patients/carers/health team.

BOX 2.4 **The SOAPC system of care**

- Subjective information: the history
- Objective information: the examination, tests, records
- Analysis: working diagnosis or differential diagnosis
- Plan: treatment and ongoing care
- Communication: with the patient, carers and other healthcare professionals

---

S – The subjective assessment

The history is the key to correct patient assessment.[13] When errors are made, they are usually attributable to inadequate history taking. It is not possible or desirable to probe every part of the patient's medical history. Instead it is important to have a system that obtains key information. A much more detailed history will be needed in the patient who is likely to be treated at home than the patient who is going to be transported to hospital. Box 2.5 sets out the main parts to history taking.

The *presenting complaint* is the main problem for the patient. When there are several presenting symptoms, choose the main problem. Explore its onset. What was the patient doing when it started? Is it getting better or worse?

Ask about *associated symptoms* relevant to the main complaint. For example, in chest pain ask about nausea, vomiting, sweating and shortness of breath. At this point ask questions relevant to the presenting complaint, for example in a patient with chest pain, ask about hypertension, diabetes and family history of heart disease.

The *history of previous episodes* may give important pointers to the diagnosis and treatment.

The *medical history* needs to be explored along with the patient's current medications. Most patients will have a list of their medications either in note form, on repeat prescription sheets, or in dispensing containers. Use these sources of information where possible.

The *social context* must be noted as this may have more bearing on the patient's future management than the diagnosis. Is there a carer who can observe the patient? Is the patient capable of performing the activities of daily life such as washing, eating, dressing and toileting?

TIP

Develop a system of appropriate history taking: 'Ask the right questions, not every question'[12]

BOX 2.5 **Main parts of history taking**

- Presenting complaint – symptoms and progress
- Associated symptoms
- Previous similar symptoms
- Previous medical problems/drug history
- Social context (including carer support, alcohol, smoking, drugs)

O – The objective assessment (examination and tests)

The most important parts of the examination can usually be performed but may be limited at the scene or in the patient's home. This inability to examine the patient properly must be taken into account when making transport, referral and treatment decisions.

As with history the examination should be targeted to the specific complaint but must always include vital signs and a general examination of the patient and their social context.

Vital signs

Pulse, blood pressure, temperature, conscious level and oxygen saturation are all easy to measure and provide objective proof of the patient's physiology at the time of the examination. Some might argue that a full set of vital signs is not required in cases of minor illness, but the situation can change and it is good practice to take baseline recordings, especially if the patient is unwell. Records of vital signs are also evidence of completion of an appropriate primary survey.

Social context

Many illnesses will be treated at home. However, in some patients, particularly elderly people living alone, even a minor illness may make extra social support a necessity. This may need help from family, carers, or even from the emergency community support team. It is important to understand the potential problems associated with the patient's immediate environment and the level of help available.

General examination

The identification of the 'unwell patient' is a prime skill of those involved in emergency medicine. There is no single sign that gives you the 'gut feeling' that the patient is ill, it is a combination of the facial appearance and the demeanour. The eyes should be checked for jaundice and pallor, the colour and perfusion of the lips and hands noted. Hydration can be assessed by checking the mucous membranes, tongue and skin turgor.

The unwell patient could have any combination of signs listed in Box 2.6.

Systems examination

In the pre-hospital setting the examination should be focused on the major presenting complaint. This may need examination of more than one system. Abnormalities in one system may lead to symptoms and signs in another part of the body. For example, an increased respiratory rate is often a sign of chest disorder but is also abnormal in diabetic ketoacidosis, shock and some poisoning.

BOX 2.6 **Some signs found in the unwell patient**

- A flat affect
- Irritability
- Pallor, sweating, and 'drawn' face
- Dark and slightly sunken eyes
- Reduced skin turgor
- A coated tongue and dry mouth
- Tachypnoea

Respiratory system

Use the *look–feel–listen* system (Box 2.7).

Look – Measure the respiratory rate and assess if the patient has any difficulty in breathing. Look for tracheal tug, the use of accessory muscles (Fig. 2.2), or in-drawing of intercostal muscles. Assess if the patient is becoming exhausted and look for excess sputum production, inhaler or home nebuliser use.

Feel – Is the chest expansion the same on both sides (Fig. 2.3)?

Listen – Check the percussion note (Fig. 2.4) and listen to the breath sounds on both sides at the apex, in the axilla and posteriorly at the top, middle and base (McGill virtual stethoscope, http://sprojects.mmi.mcgill/mvs/mvsteth.htm). The aim of auscultation is to determine whether *air entry* is normal and equal on both sides. Normal sounds are described as vesicular. If the lung is solid, sound transmission is different and the noise is similar to the sounds heard when the stethoscope is placed over the trachea (*bronchial breathing*). The next step is to assess if there are *added sounds*, these can be wheeze (inspiratory, expiratory or both) or crackles.

Function – In patients with respiratory symptoms check the oxygen saturation and in patients with asthma and other obstructive pulmonary disease check the peak expiratory flow rate.

BOX 2.7 **Summary of respiratory system examination**

■ Look at patient's lips/tongue for cyanosis
■ Measure respiratory rate
■ Assess work of breathing/dyspnoea
■ Check trachea and neck veins
■ Check chest expansion
■ Check percussion note
■ Listen to breath sounds

Fig. 2.2 The patient is gripping the arms of the chair and using neck and shoulder muscles to assist chest expansion.

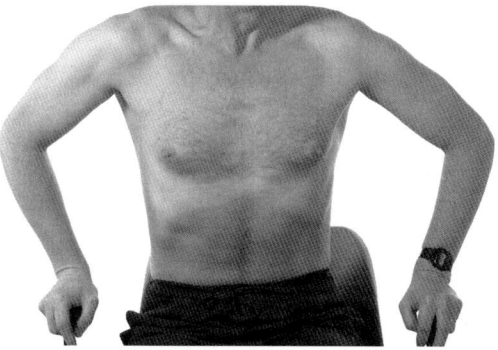

Fig. 2.3 Demonstrating chest expansion. Note the thumbs are held above the chest wall. This makes movement more obvious.

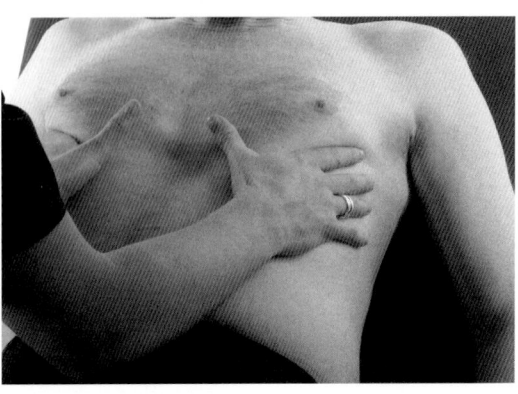

Fig. 2.4 Checking percussion note.

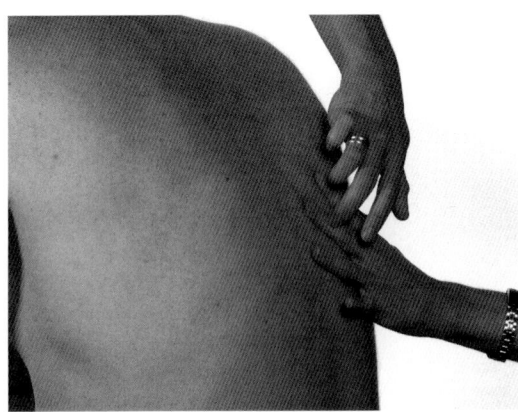

Cardiovascular system

Where the main patient complaint is not directly associated with cardiovascular abnormality, it is still good practice to screen this system. Capillary refill time, heart rate, and blood pressure would be the minimum for an ill patient.

Look – Is the patient pale? Are they sweating? Is the skin clammy? Is skin turgor normal? Look in the mouth – are the mucous membranes dry? Check the neck veins – are they full or collapsed? Check the jugular venous pulse (Fig. 2.5).

Feel – Check capillary refill time. Note the pulse rate and rhythm and character. Feel for peripheral pulses (Fig. 2.6). Look for ankle oedema. Check the calves for tenderness and swelling.

Listen – Measure the blood pressure. Listen to heart sounds (McGill virtual stethoscope) and at the lung bases for crackles (pulmonary oedema).

Fig. 2.5 Examining the jugular venous pulse. The patient is at 45°. The neck muscles are relaxed.

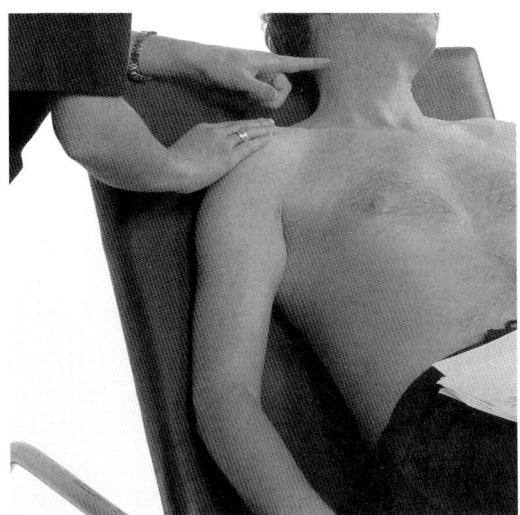

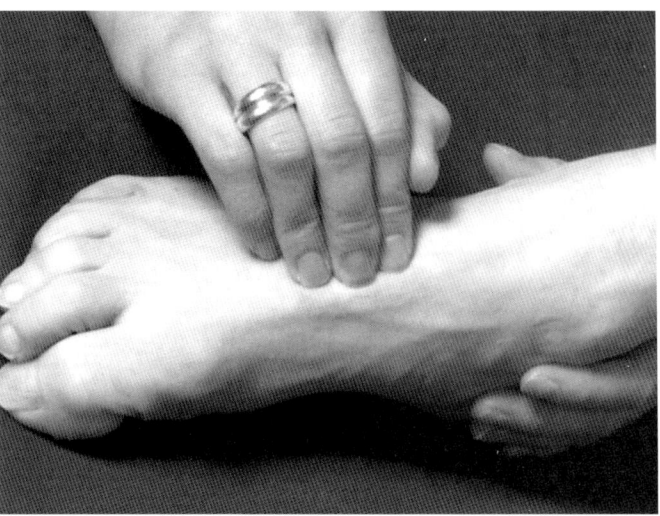

Fig. 2.6 Checking foot pulses.

Gastrointestinal system

Hydration, nutrition and looking at the mouth and tongue are part of the general examination of the patient. While examining the mouth, smell the breath. *Fetor* is a characteristic smell of the breath in a patient who is unwell. If the patient is complaining of abdominal pain the chest should also be examined.

All books of surgical examination emphasise the importance of exposing the whole abdomen, including the genitalia. In the community setting the same principle applies but it can be difficult to do this because of facilities and lack of a chaperone. If conditions do not permit a full examination then it is important to recognise that examination is incomplete. Rectal examination and vaginal examination are even more problematic. Without adequate patient consent, privacy and a chaperone these examinations should not be undertaken except in life threatening situations.

The objective of the examination is to decide if there are signs of a condition requiring hospital assessment. Signs of peritonitis, intestinal obstruction, or a vascular emergency are especially important.

The abdomen is examined using the 'look–feel–listen' system.

Look – for distension and note how the abdomen moves. Ask the patient to cough. Pain on movement and coughing is a good indicator of peritoneal irritation. Note scars and any swelling or hernias.

Feel – gently at first to try to detect any rigidity in the abdominal muscles. If there is inflammation of the peritoneum then the overlying muscles will protect the area, this is known is *guarding*. Identify the areas of maximum tenderness. Another sign of peritoneal irritation is *percussion tenderness*. Place fingers over the area of tenderness and percuss these with fingers of the other hand (Fig. 2.7). Pain during this test is indicative of peritoneal irritation.

If gentle palpation is not painful then palpate more deeply trying to find any masses. Check for enlargement of the liver and spleen. Check in the groins for swellings that might indicate a hernia (this might be quite small).

Listen – for bowel sounds. If they are absent this is a worrying finding. They may be increased in gastroenteritis but in obstruction as well as being increased they may be higher pitched or tinkling in quality.

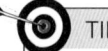

TIP

A full abdominal examination may be difficult in the patient's home, especially if there is no chaperone. If you are unable to carry out a full examination, take this into account when making treatment plans

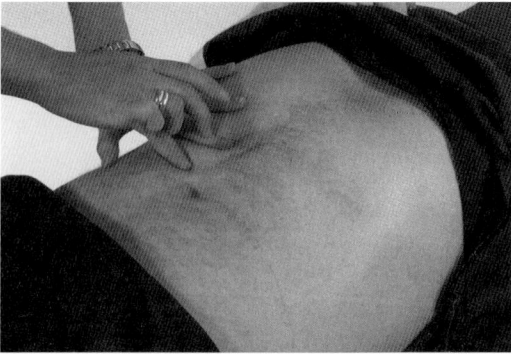

Fig. 2.7 Eliciting percussion tenderness, a good sign of peritoneal irritation.

Central nervous system screening exam

If the patient is lucid and able to give a full history and walk normally, can hold their arms out steadily with their eyes closed (Fig. 2.8), can stand on each leg with eyes closed and has normal facial expressions and eye movements there is no severe neurological deficit. This screening test is not sufficient for anyone with a primary neurological complaint.

Tests of higher mental function are a sensitive indicator of acute neurological dysfunction but they are not so specific, being very commonly affected by pre-existing problems. For example, the older patient may not be fully orientated but this may well be attributable to dementia. It is therefore important to seek information regarding the previous level of function and any change. Always take seriously a carer's view that there has been a sudden deterioration in mental function.

Record orientation in time, place and person and the Glasgow Coma Score. The Abbreviated Mental Test Score is more detailed (Box 2.8). It is especially useful in the older patient, particularly if there is access to previous records. Patients should be able to score 8/10.

The examination for the main neurological presentations can be tailored to suit the situation.

In the patient with sudden onset of headache (see 'headache' in Chapter 10) a full general examination is very important. Vital signs including pulse, blood pressure and temperature may give clues. There should be a full examination of the whole body looking for any signs of rash. Photophobia and neck stiffness should be sought (Fig. 2.9). Other signs such as muscle tenderness and Kernig's signs may be checked.

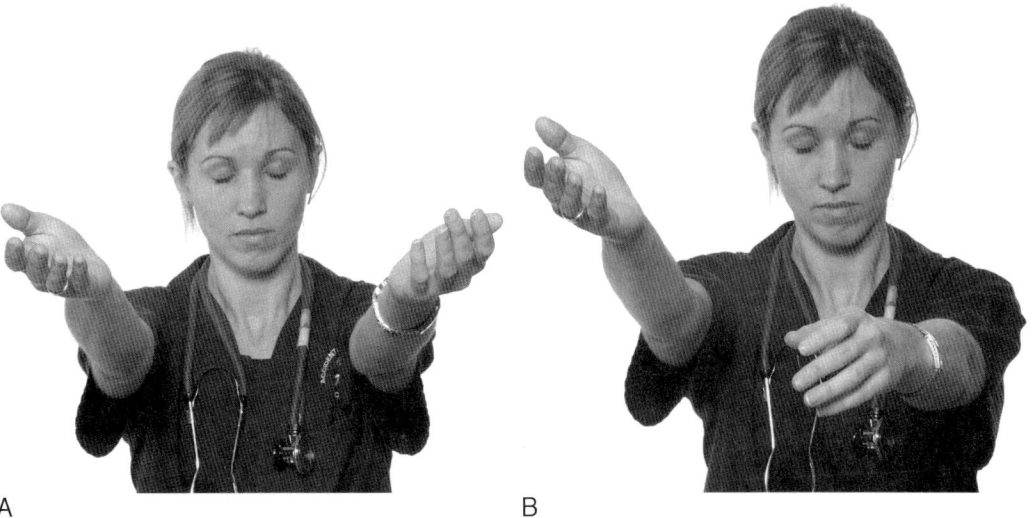

A   B

Fig. 2.8 Pronator drift. A – Ask the patient to hold arms out, palms up. B – In patients with mild limb weakness the arm drifts out and pronates (palm down).

BOX 2.8 **Abbreviated mental test score**

- Age (to exact year)
- Time (to nearest hour)
- Address recall (for example, 42 West Street)
- Year (exactly)
- Name of place (where are we)
- Recognition of two people
- Date of birth
- Queen's name
- Start of First World War (or Second World War)
- Count backwards from 20 (20, 19, 18, etc.)
- Ask for recall of address

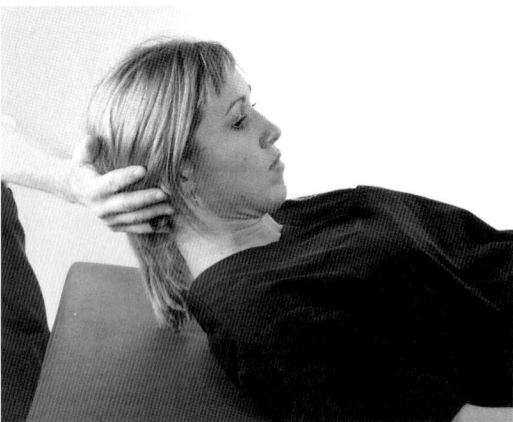

Fig. 2.9 Eliciting neck stiffness. First ask the patient to touch their chest with their chin. Note if painful. Then passively flex the neck and assess resistance. If active movement is very painful and limited, omit passive movement.

In the patient with an acute stroke, the focus will be on determining the extent of deficit and if vital functions such as airway protective reflexes are preserved.

Detailed examination of the nervous system is usually divided into testing the function of the *cranial nerves*, the nerves that provide motor and sensory function to the head and neck (or structures derived from this area of the embryo) and testing of the neurological function of the limbs.

Cranial nerve screening exam

- *CN 1* Smell not routinely tested in the emergency situation.
- *CN 2* Assessment of vision should include acuity, visual fields by confrontation (Fig. 2.10), pupillary responses, and fundoscopy when required.
- *CN 3, 4, 6* Eye movements are examined to check for diplopia.

Fig. 2.10 Visual field screening by confrontation. The patient and examiner have corresponding eyes closed and the patient looks at the examiner's nose. The patient's fields are checked against the examiner's.

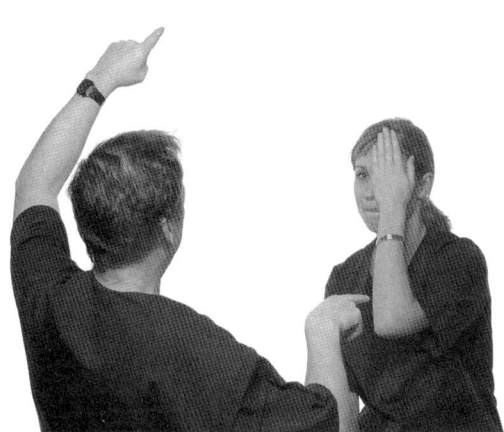

- *CN 5* Ask the patient to open the lower jaw against resistance of your hand. Check sensation over the forehead, cheeks and jaw.
- *CN 7* Look for symmetry when the patient screws up their eyes, frowns, raises eyebrows, shows their teeth, and puffs out their cheeks (Fig. 2.11).
- *CN 8* Rub fingers together gently at each ear, asking the patient if they can hear and if there is a difference between ears.
- *CN 9/10* Ask the patient to open their mouth and to say 'aah'. Assess the movement of the uvula. Check gag reflex. If there is no obvious deficit, assess swallowing by asking the patient to take a sip of water.

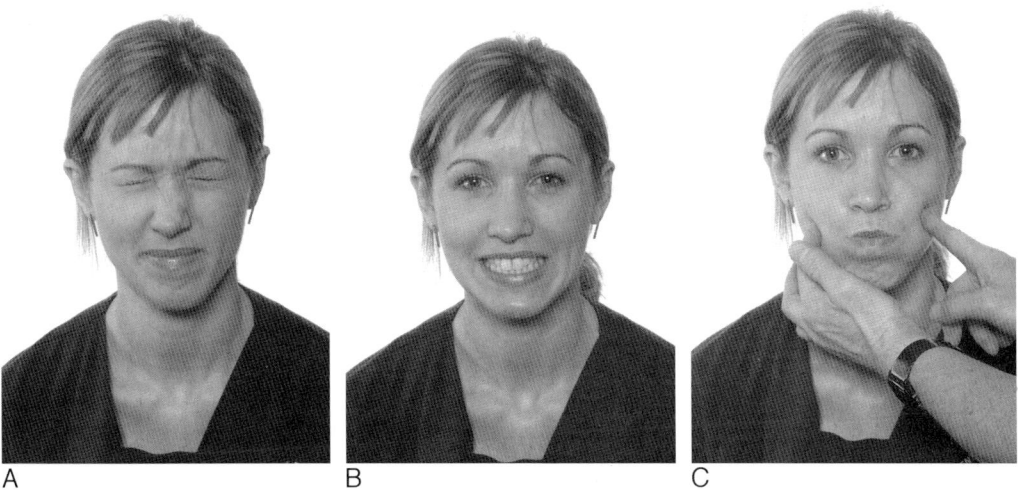

A   B   C

Fig. 2.11 Testing the CN 7 (facial nerve). A – Eye and forehead muscles. B – Muscles around the mouth. C – Cheek muscles.

- *CN 11* Ask the patient to shrug their shoulders and check the power of this movement.
- *CN 12* Ask the patient to stick their tongue out.

Peripheral nervous system exam

The objective is to assess muscle power and tone, compare sensation on each side, to check reflexes, and then to check coordination, balance, and if possible, gait.

Muscle tone is assessed by flexing and extending the elbows, wrists and knees.

Muscle power – the initial screening test for muscle power of holding out both arms is described above (see Fig. 2.8). Then assess power in the major groups acting over major joints.

Sensation – use a blunt point to assess touch (special single patient use disposable points are available). Compare sensation in both limbs. Patients may be able still to feel something even if there is a sensory deficit. You are looking for a qualitative difference in sensation (Fig. 2.12).

Reflexes are compared.

Co-ordination can be assessed by the finger–nose test (Fig. 2.13).

Balance is checked by asking the patient to stand on each leg with eyes closed. It is essential to hold the patient's hands when doing this test and it may not be possible in many patients (Fig. 2.14).

Ear, nose and throat exam

ENT examination is an integral part of the examination of the unwell adult or pyrexia of unknown origin and especially the unwell child. Check the throat and tonsils, feel the neck for lymph nodes, and check the tympanic membranes. If the patient is complaining of difficulty in swallowing, observe them drinking some water. Full details are given in Chapter 11.

Fig. 2.12 Checking sensation (sharp/blunt). Compare sensation in similar areas on each limb. You are looking for *altered* sensation.

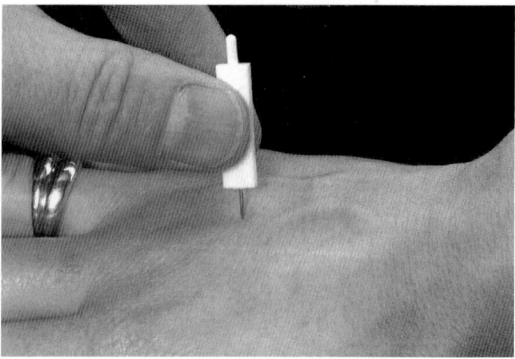

Fig. 2.13 Finger–nose test for coordination.

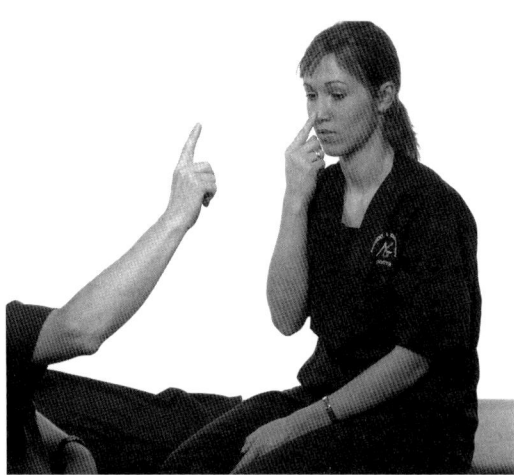

Fig. 2.14 Balancing on one leg with the eyes closed is a test of many neurological pathways including proprioception, lower limb power, balance, and the patient's general strength.

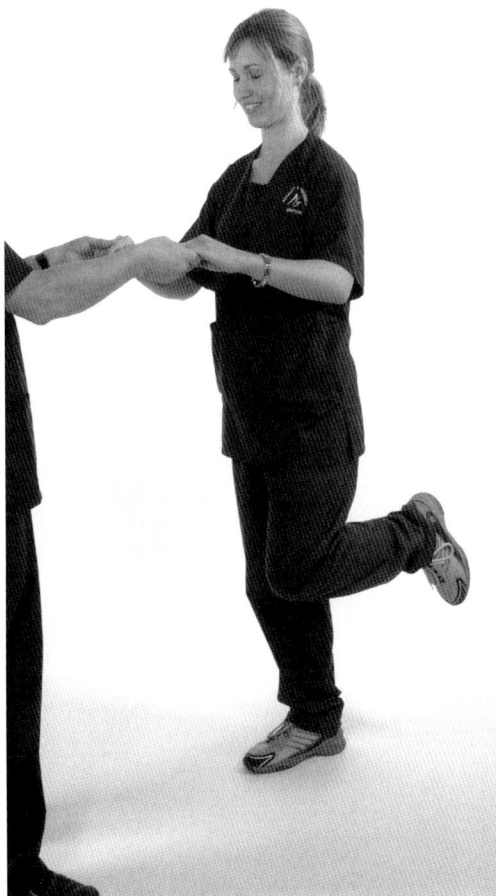

Musculoskeletal exam

The history will indicate if the problem is attributable to a recent injury or a non-traumatic problem. This is a very important distinction in a patient with musculoskeletal symptoms as the diagnostic range is very different. In the patient with no history of trauma you will need to consider if the pain is attributable to sepsis, ischaemic or vascular problems, or referred from the spine or heart/chest or abdomen.

General

In the patient with no history of injury check the temperature and pulse.

The *look–feel–move* system is used. By careful observation and palpation you can locate the *area* that has been injured, by moving it is possible to begin to decide the structure that might be injured.

Look – for swelling, bruising, redness and deformity.

Feel – palpation should start away from the most painful areas. Often checking the joint above the injury is a good way to start to gain the patient's confidence.

Movement – entails checking the active and passive *range* of the joint (limitations may indicate a joint problem). *Resisted movement* assesses muscle function and *stress testing* checks ligaments. Note function (for example, can the patient walk). Check distal nerve function and pulses.

Details of musculoskeletal examination may be found in standard texts and in Chapter 13.[14,15]

Signs of fracture include tenderness over the bone and reduction in movement. Many patients with musculoskeletal injuries will need radiography. However, where there is no deformity and no neurovascular problems the radiograph might be delayed to the most convenient time for the patient and the emergency system. Simple splints and analgesia will give you time to arrange the radiograph at the most appropriate time.

A – Analysis

Decision making and diagnosis are necessary evils. Necessary as it is not possible to decide on treatment without a working diagnosis, an evil because clinical decision making can be imprecise. A diagnosis is reached by a synthesis of the information you have. Each 'bit' of information will carry different weights. Some features, either in the history or examination, will carry so much weight that the diagnosis is easy (Fig. 2.15).

The skill of diagnosis lies firstly in eliciting the right information and secondly in the ability to 'weigh up' the evidence. This should allow you to place the patient into one of five diagnostic categories:

- Group 1: high likelihood of serious illness requiring hospital admission.

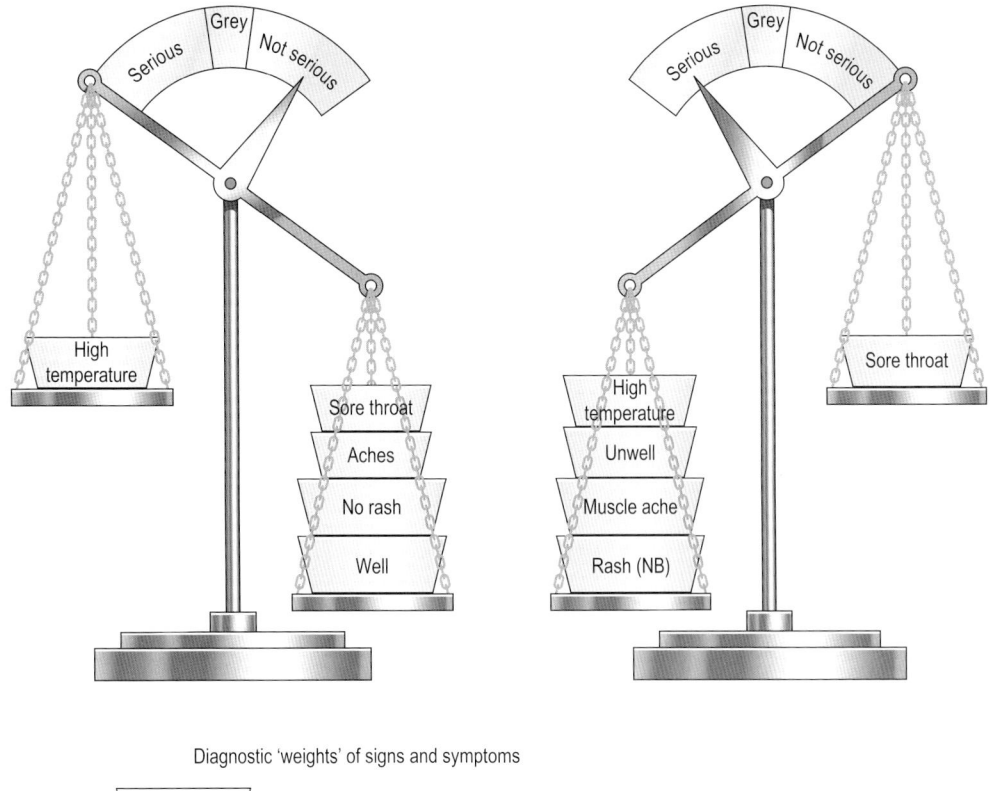

Diagnostic 'weights' of signs and symptoms

| Sore throat | Very common symptom that does not help in this diagnostic process |

| High temperature | Very common symptom that indicates a significant infection but this is commonly viral |

| Well | A very important finding that indicates low likelihood of serious illness *at this* examination |

| Non-blanching rash | A very important finding that indicates a high likelihood of serious illness. A *'red flag'* |

Fig. 2.15 Diagnostic 'weights' of signs and symptoms

- Group 2: some features or symptoms that might suggest a serious illness, needs further investigation, or a period of observation
- Group 3: high likelihood of illness that can be treated at home
- Group 4: non-specific symptoms with no signs of serious illness at present; the patient may be treated at home, with advice to seek further help if symptoms get worse
- Group 5: no evidence of a new medical condition but concern about social support and ability to cope.

If you are unsure about the diagnosis then a number of options will be available:

- refer the patient to hospital
- ask for another opinion
- seek advice over the telephone (or telemedicine link)
- give initial treatment and return within a few hours and reassess
- give initial treatment and advise the patient to seek advice if the condition does not follow the predicted course, if the symptoms get worse, or new symptoms develop.

The course of action you will take depends on the illness, the severity of possible alternative diagnoses, the patient location, your capabilities and resources, and the social context. For example, if there is uncertainty about the diagnosis in a patient with central chest pain, they should be referred or transported to hospital. Equally the young man with non-specific abdominal symptoms and signs might be best treated by active observation at home.

Investigation

There are a few investigations that are routinely available in the community. These include urine analysis, pregnancy testing, and capillary blood glucose analysis. In the future this list is likely to include near bedside testing such as cardiac troponins, D-dimers, and acute phase proteins such as C reactive protein.

P – Plan

Not every patient will fall neatly into one of the five categories listed above but this is a good framework that may guide treatment and advice.

Most patients in group 1 and group 2 will need to be taken to hospital. A few in group 2 might be observed at home, especially if advanced diagnostic facilities are available in the community. This is rare at present.

Group 3 patients will be treated at home along local guidelines and patient group directions.

Many in group 4 will be treated at home, with appropriate symptomatic treatment, and clear advice to seek further assessment if symptoms persist.

The management of patients in group 5 with social and nursing problems is difficult. Many areas now have very active community social support teams who can be called to assess the patient at home.

C – Communication

This last phase of the consultation is the most crucial part of the whole episode. Practitioners have to communicate with the patient, the carers,

---

BOX 2.9 Safety netting

- Confirm information
- Confirm understanding of treatment plans
- Ask if the patient has any questions
- Ensure they know how and when to seek further advice

---

other parts of the emergency care system, and the patient's general practitioner.

Communication with the patient and carers is vital. Check that they agree with your interpretation of the information provided. Ensure they understand your diagnosis and the treatment you are planning. Ask if they have questions. Make sure all understand what to do if the symptoms get worse or they do not improve as you predict. This process is called 'safety netting' (Box 2.9).

Communication with other parts of the healthcare system is an integral part of the emergency consultation. Making a good record of a consultation is essential. Use the same system of SOAPC to record your findings and to outline the treatment plan. The patient's general practitioner should be notified.

You may need to consult with other parts of the emergency system. A second opinion or advice should be available by telephone. Some emergency care systems may have telemedicine links.

Summary

This article has described a system of patient assessment that follows set patterns of information gathering leading to a working diagnosis. Developing and practising your own system takes time and experience. Many readers will have already developed their own methods of examination. Those who are new to clinical examination will need tuition and practice.

References

1 McQuillan P, Pilkington S, Allan A, et al 1998 Confidential inquiry into quality of care before admission to intensive care. BMJ 316:1853–1858
2 Buist M D, Moore G E, Bernard S A, et al 2002 Effects of a medical emergency team on reduction of incidence of and mortality from unexpected cardiac arrests in hospital: preliminary study. BMJ 324:387–390
3 Avery A, Pringle M 1995 Emergency care in general practice. BMJ 310:6

4   Moulds A S, Martin P B, Bouchier-Hayes T A I 1999 Emergencies in general practice, 4th edn. Librapharm, Reading
5   Sprigings D, Chambers J 2001 Acute medicine. 3rd edn. Blackwell Science, Oxford
6   Advanced Life Support Group 2001 Acute medical emergencies: the practical approach. BMJ Books, London
7   Ramrakha P, Moore K 1997 Oxford handbook of acute medicine. Oxford University Press, Oxford
8   Wyatt J P, Illingworth R N, Clancy M J, et al 1999 Oxford handbook of accident and emergency medicine. Oxford University Press, Oxford
9   Darwent M, Gregg R, Higginson I, et al 1997 What to do in a general practice emergency. BMJ Publishing Group, London
10   Greaves I, Porter K (eds) 1999 Pre-hospital medicine: the principles and practice of immediate care. Arnold, London
11   Palmer K T 1998 Notes for the MRCGP, 3rd edn. Blackwell Science, Oxford
12   Hoffbrand B I 1989 Away with the system review: a plea for parsimony. BMJ 298:817–819
13   Fraser R C 1999 The diagnostic process. In: Clinical method – a general practice approach. 3rd edn. Butterworth-Heinemann, Oxford
14   Wardrope J, English B 1998 Musculo-skeletal problems in emergency medicine. Oxford University Press, Oxford
15   McRae R 1997 Clinical orthopaedic examination. Edinburgh: Churchill Livingstone

Further reading

Clinical Method
Fraser R C (ed) 1999 Clinical method – a general practice approach, 3rd edn. Butterworth-Heinemann, Oxford
Munro J F, Campbell I W 2000 MacLeod's clinical examination, 10th edn. Churchill Livingstone, Edinburgh

Differential Diagnosis
Bouchier I A D, Ellis H, Fleming P R 1996 French's index of differential diagnosis, 13th edn. Butterworth-Heinemann, Oxford
Hopcroft K, Forte V 1999 Symptom sorter. Radcliffe Medical Press, Oxford
Seller R H 2000 Differential diagnosis of common complaints, 4th edn. WB Saunders, Pennsylvania
Taylor R B 2000 The ten minute diagnosis manual. Lippincott Williams, Philadelphia

Colville Laird, Peter Driscoll and Jim Wardrope

Chest pain

Introduction

Chest pain is the commonest reason for 999 calls and accounts for 2.5% of out-of-hours calls. Of patients taken to hospital, about 10% will have an acute myocardial infarction (AMI). Evidence suggests that up to 7.5% of these will be missed on first presentation. There are a number of other life threatening conditions which can present as chest pain and must not be overlooked. The objectives of this article are therefore to provide a safe and comprehensive system of dealing with this presenting complaint (Box 3.1).

> **BOX 3.1 Objectives of assessment of patients with chest pain**
>
> - To undertake a primary survey of the patient and treat any immediately life threatening problems
> - To identify any patients who have a normal primary survey but have an obvious need for hospital admission
> - To undertake a secondary survey considering other systems of the body where dysfunction could present as chest pain
> - To consider a list of differential diagnoses
> - Discuss treatment based on the probable diagnosis(es) and whether home management or hospital admission is appropriate
> - Consider follow up if not admitted

Primary survey

Follow the ABC principles (Box 3.2).

> **BOX 3.2 Primary survey**
>
> If any of the following present treat immediately and transfer to hospital:
> - airway obstruction
> - respiratory rate <10 or >29 per minute
> - O_2 saturation <93%
> - pulse <50 or >120
> - systolic BP <90 mmHg
> - Glasgow coma score <12

Patients with normal primary survey with obvious need for hospital admission

There are three immediately life threatening medical conditions that can present with chest pain:

- acute coronary syndrome (ACS)
- pulmonary embolus
- dissection of the thoracic aorta.

The history and a brief examination may lead you to suspect that one of these is the probable diagnosis. Patients may often have normal physical signs. Urgent hospital admission must be arranged if you suspect any of the above or any other life threatening diagnosis.

Fifty percent of sudden cardiac deaths occur within 1 hour of the start of a myocardial infarction and 75% within 3 hours. The benefits of thrombolysis or percutaneous intervention (PCI) are directly related to the length of time between the onset of symptoms and its delivery. Therefore if you diagnose a myocardial infarction, ensure you have immediate access to a defibrillator and consider thrombolysis or arrange rapid transportation to a facility where thrombolysis or PCI can be delivered.

Secondary survey (including history taking)

Having dealt with the potential life threatening cases you will be left with a group of patients for whom a more thorough clinical examination will be required before considering whether they can be either treated and left at home, or referred elsewhere.

Take a history of the presenting complaint, gather relevant information, and perform an examination (see Chapter 2).

For patients with chest pain, respiratory, cardiovascular, abdominal and musculoskeletal examinations are appropriate.

There is good evidence that history and examination cannot 'rule out' any specific diagnosis, especially acute myocardial infarction. Some types of pain are more commonly found in patients with ischaemia. However there is good evidence that history can help 'risk stratify' patients. In the context of acute chest pain, some other investigation will often be required.

The OPQRST of chest pain

Chest pain is often categorised into three main types (Table 3.1). It can be very difficult to place any particular patient into one of these categories, but there is evidence that the characteristics of pain can help in the diagnosis:

- typical cardiac pain
- pleuritic chest pain
- atypical chest pain.

Somatic pain may arise from the chest wall (skin, ribs and intercostal muscles), pericardium (fibrous and parietal layer), and the parietal pleura. Pain from these structures is transmitted to the brain by the somatic nerve fibres that enable the brain to accurately locate the site of the problem. In the case of pleuritic chest pain, it will also be specifically related to movements of breathing.

Visceral pain in contrast originates from the deeper thoracic structures (heart, blood vessels and oesophagus) and is carried in the autonomic nerve fibres. These give a less precise location of the pain, and the pain is generally described as a discomfort, heaviness or ache. It is often referred to shoulders, arm or jaw.

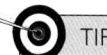 TIP

Always ask about the relation of the pain to breathing, movement, exercise and rest

TABLE 3.1 The three main types of chest pain			
	Typical ischaemic	Typical pleuritic	Atypical
Onset	Usually acute over a few minutes, but may be gradual. May be retrosternal burning	Sudden in PE pneumothorax and sometimes with infection. Gradual infection	Often vague, 'indigestion'
Precipitating or palliative factors	Worse with exercise, better with GTN or rest. Pain at rest worrying	Worse on deep breathing, coughing	Can be improved by antacids but so might pain from ACS
Quality	Tight squeezing	Sharp	Ache, fullness
Radiation	Shoulders, arm, jaw, back	Shoulder if diaphragm involved	Epigastrium
Systemic symptoms	Sweating, nausea, vomiting, SOB	Sweating, SOB, cough sputum	
Timing	Worse with exercise, rest pain or pain at night – red flag		May be related to food
Main differential	Angina (stable), acute coronary syndrome (including unstable angina), myocardial infarct	Pneumonia, pneumothorax, pulmonary embolism, viral infection	Acute coronary syndrome, GORD, non-specific chest pain

Onset of pain

The pain of a myocardial infarction is classically described as rapidly increasing over a few minutes but it can develop gradually or even be intermittent. In an acute coronary syndrome the pain may well be intermittent. As the platelet thrombus breaks down, blood flow is restored and the pain is relieved. Beware of pain starting at rest, or that which wakes the patient up from sleep.

Precipitating factors/palliative factors

Gain a detailed impression of how the pain started. Establish if there is any relation to exercise, breathing or food. Pain that has been provoked by exercise or wakened the patient should be regarded as significant. GTN will improve angina pain but also will improve pain from oesophageal problems. Equally there is no evidence that improvement of pain after giving an antacid can help distinguish between cardiac and oesophageal pain.

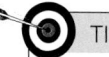

TIP

The pain due to ACS may be intermittent and *appear* to be responsive to antacids

Quality

Typical myocardial pain is easily recognised. It is often described as tight or squeezing. In a typical myocardial infarct it is very severe. Typical pleuritic pain is sharper and well localised. Atypical pain can take any form but is often described as 'indigestion' or retro-sternal burning. Such pain is also associated with inferior ischaemia and infarction.

Radiation and systemic symptoms

Typical ischaemic pain is often across the chest with radiation to the shoulders, arms or jaw. However it can be felt only in the jaw, arms, shoulder or back, or epigastrium. Pleuritic pain is well localised although it may be referred to the shoulder if the diaphragm is irritated.

Sweating, nausea, vomiting and shortness of breath are common in severe myocardial ischaemia. Ask about cough and sputum production. If the pain is pleuritic, ask about leg swelling or pain.

Timing

Typical cardiac pain that lasts less than 15 minutes is defined as angina; however, if the angina pain is of recent onset, occurring at rest, coming more often than the patient's usual angina or if it lasts more than 15 minutes, this could indicate an acute coronary syndrome (unstable angina). It would be unusual for it to continue for over 24 hours. Chest pain lasting only a few seconds is unlikely to be cardiac.

Other factors

Previous similar symptoms

A previous history of ischemic heart disease makes it much more probable that the pain is cardiac. However, patients with heart disease do have other chest problems and the patient may say that the pain is different from the usual symptoms.

Risk factors

The presence of risk factors for cardiovascular disease should increase your suspicion as to a cardiac cause for the pain (Box 3.3).

> **BOX 3.3 Important risk factors for angina or acute coronary syndrome**
>
> - Previous history of ischaemic heart disease
> - Smoking
> - Hypertension
> - Diabetes
> - Strong family history (that is, ischaemic heart disease onset <60 years)
> - High cholesterol concentrations

Medical history/drugs allergies

It is important during the history taking to ask the patient about their medical history as they may already have had an illness that could present as chest pain. A drug history is also important; specifically ask about aspirin (you may need to give this), and if they have taken GTN, warfarin, or other cardiac medications.

TIMI scoring

TIMI risk scoring is one method of assessing the risk of a patient of having a significant cardiac event (MI, death, need for revascularisation) within the next 2 weeks. It assesses seven variables listed in Box 3.4. Cardiac markers are not routinely available at present in the community setting. If a patient has no or only one point the risk of an event is 4.7% (note even this is an appreciable risk). If they have 6 points the risk is 40%. While TIMI scoring can be used to guide therapy in the hospital setting it should not be used to 'rule out' ischaemic heart disease in the community setting.

> **BOX 3.4 TIMI scoring**
>
> TIMI risk scoring assesses seven variables:
> - age > 65 years
> - at least three risk factors for cardiac disease
> - known coronary stenosis of 50% or more
> - ST segment changes on the ECG
> - at least two anginal events in the previous 24 hours
> - use of aspirin in the last 7 days
> - elevated cardiac markers
>   TIMI scoring: risk of events in 14 days – score 0–1 = 4%, 2 = 8%, 3 = 13%, 4 = 19%, 5 = 26%, 6 or 7 = 41% (see Antman et al 2000)

Social history and substances

Some illegal drugs such as cocaine may cause chest pain. Patients with a history of alcohol misuse or illegal drug use are at increased risk of developing chest infections and suffering from thromboembolic disease.

Examination

See Chapter 2 for a full discussion of examination techniques.

Vital signs

Unless you are transporting the patient immediately, always measure a full set of vital signs.

General

Is the patient confused/anxious, short of breath? This may indicate a critical situation. Go back to primary survey.

Is the patient obviously in pain? Are they pale/sweaty? Have they been sick? If the answer to any of these questions is positive, there is a greater likelihood of serious disease.

Cardiovascular

Pay special attention to the rate and rhythm of the arterial pulse and the level of the jugular venous pulse. Ask the patient to take a deep breath, look for an increase in pain during inspiration. Follow this by listening to the heart sounds and the lung bases. Finish by examining the ankles, calves and foot pulses (for oedema/signs of DVT).

Chest wall tenderness reproducing the patient's pain is suggestive of musculoskeletal pain but studies have shown this sign to be present in up to 15% of patients with confirmed myocardial infarction. Therefore this sign on its own should never be used to exclude a myocardial infarction.

Tests

An ECG is indicated in patients with chest pain. Under the age of 30, ischaemic heart disease is uncommon but if the pain is typical, obtain a 12-lead ECG. Detailed interpretation of the ECG is beyond the scope of this chapter but readers are referred to the texts in the further reading list. An abnormal ECG in a patient with chest pain is an indication for admission to hospital.

Differential diagnosis

Table 3.2 shows a list of the differential diagnoses classified by the type of pain they present with.

TABLE 3.2 Differential diagnoses		
Cardiac ischaemic pain	Pleuritic pain	Atypical pain
Angina	Pneumonia	Non-specific chest pain
Acute coronary syndrome	Pulmonary embolism	Oesophageal pain
(Dissecting aortic aneurysm)	Pneumothorax	Cardiac pain
(Oesophageal pain)	Rib injury	Gastric/biliary pain
(Pericarditis)	(Pericarditis)	Chest wall pain
		Pericarditis
		Dissecting aortic aneurysm

Cardiac pain

Ischaemic cardiac pain originates from the myocardium when its blood supply is insufficient for its needs. It can be broadly divided into two categories – angina and acute coronary syndrome.

Angina is arbitrarily defined as lasting less than 15 minutes. It is often related to increased myocardial oxygen demand, for example, stress or exercise. If angina is of recent onset, occurring at rest, increasing in frequency or lasting more than 15 minutes, acute coronary syndrome needs to be excluded. Acute coronary syndrome includes:

- infarction with ST elevation (STEMI) – usually progresses to Q wave MI (QMI)
- MI confirmed but no Q developed (NQMI) – usually no ST elevation either (NSTEMI)
- MI occurring with left bundle branch block (LBBB) hiding ST elevation
- ACS *without* serological evidence of MI (unstable angina).

Chest pain

Table 3.3 provides a summary of causes and types of chest pain.

Angina

Consider this diagnosis if the pain lasted less than 15 minutes or settles within 5 minutes of GTN administration and is a single episode. If it occurs at rest or is more severe than the patient's usual angina, consider

TABLE 3.3 Summary of causes and types of chest pain

Aetiology	Type of pain	Site of pain	Radiation	Duration of pain	Associated symptoms	Mode of onset	ECG findings	Risk factors
Angina	Visceral	Retrosternal	Neck, jaw, shoulder and arm	>15 min	Nausea and dyspnoea	Variable	ST elevation or depression	
Pericarditis	Somatic	Midline	Neck, back or shoulder	Hours to days	Pain worse on movement or breathing	Variable	ST elevation in all leads except aVR and V1	Viral infection, recent MI trauma, post-cardiac surgery
Dissecting aortic aneurysm	Visceral, severe	Retrosternal	Interscapular	Variable	Nausea and breathlessness	Sudden	Non-specific	History of hypertension
Cervical nerve root pain	Sharp or aching, superficial	Upper chest – possibly one sided	Neck	Variable	May be exacerbated by neck movement	Variable	None	
Chest wall pain	Sharp or aching	Localised	None	Variable	None	Variable	None	
Pneumothorax	Pleuritic	Usually lateral aspect of chest wall	Neck and back	Variable	Breathlessness	Sudden	None	COPD, trauma, tall, thin, young people
Pulmonary embolism	Pleuritic	Usually lateral aspect of chest wall	None	Variable	Breathlessness, unilateral swollen leg	Sudden	Non-specific ST changes, tachycardia	Recent trauma or surgery, venous stasis or hypercoagulability
Infection	Pleuritic or somatic	Usually lateral aspect of chest wall	None	Variable	Breathlessness, bronchi, bronchial breathing	Variable	None	URTI, cough, sputum, fever
Oesophageal pain	Aching or burning	Retrosternal	Interscapular	Minutes to hours	Difficulty or pain on swallowing	Variable	None	Gastro-oesophageal reflux disease

it to be acute coronary syndrome and refer. If the patient is young (35–70) and this is the first episode of typical ischaemic pain and has come on at rest, refer even with one episode.

Myocardial infarction

Carry out a full ABC assessment and provide oxygen and analgesia (appropriate to the diagnosis). A defibrillator must be taken to any patient complaining of chest pain. See Box 3.5 for the management of MI.

Who can be left at home?

Consider this option if the patient has a history of angina, and they have had a typical episode lasting less than 15 minutes, they are well and the ECG is normal. They must of course be told to call for assistance if the pain recurs. It is desirable to have a relative or carer stay with them, or to do a check by visit or telephone in a few hours.

Pericarditis

The pericardium is a double layer of tissue, which envelops the heart. It has an outer thick, fibrous layer that is attached to the base of the great vessels and the diaphragm. The gap between the heart and this fibrous layer is called the pericardial space. This is covered by a thin, serous

---

BOX 3.5 JRCALC MI management

- Administer 400 µg GTN where systolic BP is estimated >90 mmHg
- Give high flow oxygen via a non-rebreathing mask
- Where appropriate move to the ambulance at this stage
- If pain persists consider a second dose of 400 µg GTN where systolic BP is estimated >90 mmHg
- Give aspirin 300 mg orally
- Obtain intravenous access if not already achieved
- Monitor BP for hypotension and position patient appropriately
- If pain continues, morphine 2.5–10 mg intravenously may be administered
- Pain assessment scoring should be carried out before and after analgesia has been administered
- **Remove to nearest suitable receiving hospital without delay for urgent thrombolytic therapy**
  If trained in thrombolysis then:
- ensure the patient has the indications (typical chest pain + appropriate ST elevation; LBBB)
- ensure the patient has no contraindications
- explain risks and benefits
- obtain consent and administer thrombolysis

layer, which lines the inner surface of the fibrous pericardium as well as the outer surface of the heart. Normally the two serous layers slide over one another during the movement of the heart, an action facilitated by the small amount of fluid in pericardial space. However, in pericarditis the surfaces become swollen, tender and inflamed. This usually results from infection but it can result from autoimmune reactions, after myocardial infarction and cardiac surgery. Pericarditis commonly presents as chest pain described as midline and sharp. The pain is made worse by movement and breathing, whereas sitting up and leaning forward may relieve it. The pain may radiate to the back, neck or left shoulder and is associated with dyspnoea, tiredness and fever.

Dissecting aortic aneurysm

In this condition blood breaks through the inner lining of the aorta and creates a false passage between the endothelium and the outer wall. In doing so it may occlude the branches of the aorta and give rise to a variety of conditions including strokes. It may also track proximally and burst through into the pericardium or damage the aortic valve. One of the signs of this can be disparity between the upper limb blood pressure recordings.

Typically the patient presents with severe, 'ripping/sharp' chest pain radiating through to the back. Diagnosis is difficult but is made easier by thinking of the condition, particularly in those with a higher risk (for example, hypertension or Marfan's syndrome). Examination may reveal a difference in the blood pressure between the left and right arm. There may be murmurs heard over the back.

Patients with ACS, pericarditis or thoracic aortic dissection will usually have had problems identified in the primary survey. If not, correct any ABC abnormality, give pain relief and arrange immediate admission to hospital.

Cervical root pain

This occurs when one of the nerves that exits the cervical spine is irritated by structures within the vertebral column. The pain is limited to the upper chest and the neck and is usually precipitated by neck movement. These patients will not normally require admission. Treatment will be from the following options: analgesia, non-steroidal anti-inflammatory drugs, muscle relaxants, and a soft cervical collar.

Chest wall pain

This is pain originating from the ribs or chest wall musculature, or both. It may be related to trauma, in which case the area of tenderness is at the site of injury. In non-trauma cases, the pain and tenderness are usually over the anterior chest wall. Treatment is with non-steroidal anti-inflammatory drugs. If associated with major trauma, patients should be admitted.

Pneumothorax

A pneumothorax is the complete or partial collapse of a lung. There is usually a sudden onset of sharp chest pain and dyspnoea. The pain is normally one sided and may radiate to the back. Risk factors include obstructive pulmonary disease, trauma and tall thin young people. Treat any ABC abnormality and provide oxygen and analgesia. This patient will need to be sent to hospital.

Pulmonary embolism

This occurs when a clot forms within the venous system of the body and then travels to the lungs and obstructs part of the pulmonary circulation. The onset of symptoms is sudden, often unilateral and associated with dyspnoea and tachypnoea (respiratory rate >20).

Risk factors include intravenous drug abuse, a recent history of trauma or surgery, venous stasis or hypercoagulability. The pre-test probability of a pulmonary embolism can be predicted from Table 3.4.

The vital signs may be abnormal and hence the patient will be primary survey positive. If this is not the case, but pulmonary embolism is suspected, appropriate resuscitation should be started, if required, and the patient sent to hospital.

TABLE 3.4 Pre-test probability of pulmonary embolism well's criteria	
Factor	Risk score
Clinical signs of DVT	3.0
Other diagnosis less likely	3.0
HR >100	1.5
Stasis or operation in <4/52	1.5
History of DVT or PE	1.5
Active Ca or treatment in <6/12	1.0
Haemoptysis	1.0
Low risk 2 or less; moderate risk 2–6; high risk > 6.	

Infection

The patient may have a history of a current or recent upper respiratory tract infection and a productive cough. On examination there may also be fever and breathlessness. To make decisions on treatment and whether the patient can be left at home, the following guidelines from the British Thoracic Society should be used – admit if:

■ Children
 – Oxygen saturation <92%
 – Respiratory rate >50 breath/min, under 1 year 70 breath/min
 – Difficulty in breathing
 – Grunting
 – Signs of dehydration
 – Family not able to provide appropriate observation and supervision
 – Unable to take antibiotics because of vomiting

■ Adults
 – Confused
 – Oxygen saturation <92%
 – Respiratory rate >30 breath/min
 – Low blood pressure (systolic <90 mmHg, diastolic < 60 mmHg)
 – >50 years of age or have co-existing disease
 – Unable to take antibiotics because of vomiting.

Treatment

If admission is not planned encourage the patient to rest, drink plenty of fluids and not to smoke. Pleuritic pain should be treated with simple analgesics.

Amoxicillin is the antibiotic of choice for adults, with erythromycin or clarithromycin as an alternative for patients who are hypersensitive to penicillins.

All children under 1 year should be examined by a doctor. Amoxicillin is the first choice of antibiotic for children under 5. Alternatives are co-amoxiclav, cefaclor, erythromycin, clarithromycin and azithromycin.

In children over 5, erythromycin or clarithromycin may be used as a first line treatment as mycoplasma pneumonia is more prevalent in this older age group.

Arrange review within 24 to 48 hours.

Oesophageal pain

This pain is caused by acid reflux from the stomach burning the oesophageal mucosa. The pain may be of variable onset relieved by antacids, burning in nature, radiate to between the shoulder blades, and be accompanied by swallowing difficulties. Pain may be related to eating. Beware that acute coronary syndrome may present with 'indigestion' or retrosternal burning.

Treatment is with antacids, H2 antagonists, or proton pump inhibitors. If it does not respond to treatment, or swallowing difficulties develop, the patient should be admitted.

Beware of labelling pain as oesophageal or chest wall pain unless you have specific reasons that support this diagnosis.

 PITFALLS

It is important to remember that oesophageal pain may be relieved with GTN and that some anginal pain may appear to be relieved by antacids. This is especially true of acute coronary syndrome where the pain may well be intermittent and appears to 'settle'.

Diagnoses for exclusion

Undertaking all of the above steps will help you reach a diagnosis. It is vital to appreciate that included in the differential diagnosis are:

- acute coronary syndrome
- pulmonary embolism
- dissection of the thoracic aorta
- pneumothorax.

Interpretation of findings

These conditions require the patient to be admitted to hospital as soon as possible so it is important that these conditions are not missed. Thus if a convincing diagnosis of a condition other than these four cannot be reached the patient should be admitted to hospital. Individual symptoms or signs are unreliable (for example, there is no guarantee that a somatic pain is not originating from the heart or that heart pain will not disappear after the administration of an antacid). It is therefore unwise to exclude the diagnosis based on a single symptom, physical sign or investigation. Instead it should be based on several supporting pieces of information.

Treatment and disposal

- *Treat and Refer* – ACS, dissecting aortic aneurysm, pleuritic chest pain (depending on diagnosis and condition of patient), pneumothorax, gastrointestinal pain (depending on condition of patient or not settling with appropriate treatment)

■ *Treat and Leave* – stable angina, cervical root pain, chest wall pain, pleuritic chest pain (depending on diagnosis and condition of patient), gastrointestinal pain (depending on condition of patient or not settling with appropriate treatment).

Follow-up arrangements (if not admitted)

Arrange review if indicated before normal working hours or, if not, notify the responsible GP with appropriate information at the start of normal working hours.

Further reading

Diagnosis

Antman E M, Cohen M, Bernick P J L M et al 2000 The TIMI Risk Score for unstable angina/non ST elevation MI. JAMA 284:835–842

Klompas M 2002 Does this patient have an acute thoracic aortic dissection? JAMA 287:2262–2272

Panju A A, Hemmelgarn B R, Guyatt G H et al 1998 Is this patient having a myocardial infarction? JAMA 280:1256–1263

Swap C J, Nagurney J T 2005 Value and limitations of chest pain history in the evaluation of patients with suspected acute coronary syndromes. JAMA 294:2623–2629

ECG Interpretation

Channer K, Morris F 2002 ABC of clinical electrocardiography: myocardial ischaemia. BMJ 324:1023–1036. Available online: http://bmj.bmjjournals. com/cgi/content/full/324/7344/1023?eaf (5 Mar 2007)

Foster B 1996 12-Lead electrocardiography for ACLS providers. WB Saunders, Philadelphia

Meek S, Morris F 2002 ABC of clinical electrocardiography: introduction. I – Leads, rate, rhythm, and cardiac axis. BMJ 324:415–418. Available online: http://bmj.bmjjournals.com/cgi/content/full/324/7334/415 (5 Mar 2007)

Meek S, Morris F 2002 ABC of clinical electrocardiography: introduction. II – Basic terminology. BMJ 324:470–473. Available online: http://bmj. bmjjournals.com/cgi/content/full/324/7335/470?eaf (5 Mar 2007)

Meek S, Morris F 2002 ABC of clinical electrocardiography: acute myocardial infarction – part II. BMJ 324:963–966. Available online: http://bmj. bmjjournals.com/cgi/content/full/324/7343/963?eaf (5 Mar 2007)

Morris F, Brady W J 2002 ABC of clinical electrocardiography: acute myocardial infarction – Part I. BMJ 324:831–834. Available online: http://bmj. bmjjournals.com/cgi/content/full/324/7341/831?eaf (5 Mar 2007)

Heart and Lung Sounds

Auscultation Assistant – http://www.med.ucla.edu/wilkes/intro.html (5 Mar 2007)

Treatment

Boehringer Ingelheim 2003 Thrombolysis up front version 2.2, May 2003. Boehringer Ingelheim, Bracknell

British Thoracic Society 2001 Guidelines for the management of community acquired pneumonia in adults. Thorax 56(suppl 4):1–64

British Thoracic Society 2002 Guidelines for the management of community acquired pneumonia in childhood. Thorax 57(suppl 1):1–24

Joint Royal Colleges Ambulance Liaison Committee 2002 Guidelines version 2. JRCALC Royal College of Physicians, London Available online: http://www.asancep.org.uk/JRCALC/guidelines.htm (5 Mar 2007)

Malcolm Woollard and Ian Greaves

Shortness of breath

Introduction

Shortness of breath is the chief complaint in approximately 8% of 999 calls to the ambulance service, and is the third most common type of emergency call. It can also be an important symptom in patients with a wide range of conditions. Reference should therefore be made to other relevant chapters – particularly that discussing chest pain (Chapter 3). The conditions covered in this chapter include asthma, chronic obstructive pulmonary disease, acute pulmonary oedema and chest infections. The objectives are listed in Box 4.1.

The common causes of shortness of breath are asthma, chronic obstructive pulmonary disease and pulmonary oedema but there are many other conditions that can pose diagnostic problems (Box 4.2).

BOX 4.1 Chapter objectives

- To consider the causes of breathlessness
- To describe the recognition of primary survey positive patients and treatment of immediately life threatening problems
- To describe the recognition and treatment of primary survey negative patients requiring immediate hospital admission
- To describe the findings and treatment of primary survey negative patients suggesting delayed admission, treatment and referral, or treatment and discharge may be appropriate

---

BOX 4.2 Causes of breathlessness

Very common
- Asthma
- Chronic obstructive pulmonary disease (COPD)
- Pulmonary oedema due to left ventricular failure

Common
- Pneumonia
- Pneumothorax
- Pulmonary embolus
- Pleural effusion
- Pregnancy

Rare
- Metabolic acidosis
- Aspirin poisoning
- Renal failure

Primary survey positive patients

Recognition

Patients with a life threatening respiratory emergency will present in either respiratory failure or respiratory distress. Patients with respiratory distress are still able to compensate for the effects of their illness, and urgent treatment may prevent their further deterioration. They present with signs and symptoms indicating increased work of breathing but findings suggesting systemic effects of hypoxia or hypercapnia will be limited or absent. Conversely, patients with respiratory failure may have limited evidence of increased work of breathing as they become too exhausted to compensate. The systemic effects of hypoxia and hypercapnia will be particularly evident in this group and immediate treatment will be required to prevent cardiac arrest. The key findings of primary survey positive patients with shortness of breath are presented in Box 4.3.

 PITFALL

Cessation of wheeze in a patient with severe asthma may be misinterpreted as an improvement in the patient's condition

TIP

Cyanosis may be detected in patients with increased skin pigmentation by examining the inside of the mouth and eyelids

---

BOX 4.3 Recognition of the primary survey positive patient with shortness of breath

Increased work of breathing
- Stridor associated with other key findings
- Use of accessory muscles
- Need to sit upright
- Tracheal tug
- Intercostal recession
- Expiratory wheeze associated with other key findings
- Cessation of expiratory wheeze without improvement in condition
- Inability to speak in whole sentences

Systemic effects of inadequate respiration
- Respiratory rate <10 or >29
- Weak respiratory effort
- Decreased, asymmetrical, or absent breath sounds
- Oxygen saturation <92% on air or <95% on high concentration oxygen
- PEFR < 33% of normal
- Hypercapnia (measured with end-tidal CO_2 monitor)
- Tachycardia ≥120 or bradycardia (late and ominous finding)
- Dysrhythmias
- Pallor and/or cyanosis (particularly central cyanosis)
- Cool clammy skin
- Falling blood pressure (late and ominous finding)
- Altered mental status – confusion, feeling of impending doom, combativeness
- Falling level of consciousness
- Exhaustion (± muscular chest pain)

Treatment

If it is not possible to obtain an airway, if the patient's condition is deteriorating rapidly, or they show signs of significant respiratory failure (in particular failure to maintain SpO_2 of 95% on high concentration oxygen) consider immediate transportation to a hospital with appropriate facilities. Important treatment points for primary survey positive patients are listed in Box 4.4.

BOX 4.4 Treatment for primary survey positive patients

Treatment before transportation
1. Secure the airway (in moribund patients it may be necessary to escalate rapidly through manual methods, simple adjuncts, intubation, and cricothyroidotomy until airway secured)
2. High concentration oxygen via non-rebreathing mask (consider titrating concentration to a COPD patient's 'normal' SpO_2)[1]
3. Assist ventilations if respiratory rate <10 or >29, titrated to SpO_2
4. Nebulised beta-2 agonist in the presence of wheeze (e.g. salbutamol 5 mg initially)
5. Nebulised anticholinergic in the presence of asthma or COPD (e.g. ipratropium bromide 0.5 mg, may be mixed with salbutamol)
6. IM epinephrine in the presence of anaphylaxis
7. Decompress tension pneumothorax
8. Consider MI/acute coronary syndrome: if present consider nitrates, aspirin, and morphine as well as thrombolysis and heparinisation (see Chapter 3)

Treatment during transportation
In addition to the above, consider:
1. Further nebulised beta-2 bronchodilators (no maximum dose for salbutamol)
2. IV fluids (asthma and anaphylaxis)
3. Intravenous or oral steroids (asthma and anaphylaxis)
4. Anti-histamines (anaphylaxis)

Primary survey negative patients with need for hospital attendance

Primary survey negative patients with the findings listed in Box 4.5 who do not respond to pre-hospital treatment will require hospital admission.

Fig. 4.1 Improvised large volume spacer using plastic soft drinks bottle

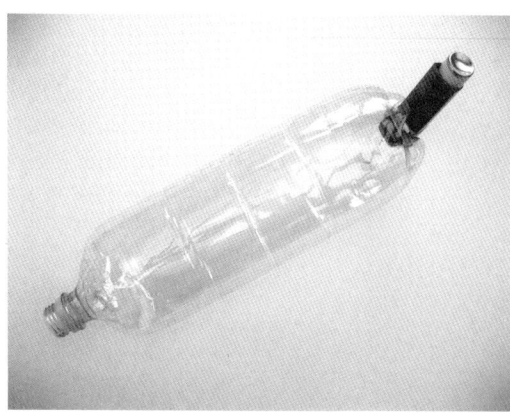

BOX 4.5 Diagnostic criteria for primary survey negative patients requiring hospital admission

Findings (not reversed by initial treatment) suggesting need for hospital admission:

- Inspiratory or expiratory noises (stridor or wheeze) audible without the aid of a stethoscope
- Cannot speak in whole sentences
- Respiration ≥25 breaths per minute
- Pulse ≥110 beats per minutes
- Supplemental oxygen required to maintain SpO_2 at 95% or above (or at 'usual' level of SpO_2 for COPD patients)
- PEFR <50% of normal
- Inability to rule out MI or acute coronary syndrome
- Lack of carer support for those patients unable to look after themselves

---

Secondary survey

The SOAPC system should be used to undertake a secondary survey (see Chapter 2). In primary survey positive patients, a secondary survey may not be completed in the pre-hospital phase of treatment as the focus must be on treatment of life threatening problems. For primary survey negative patients requiring hospital care the secondary survey may be undertaken during transportation. For the remaining patient population a secondary survey may be undertaken at the point of contact and will contribute to the decision to admit, treat and refer, or treat and leave.

Subjective assessment

Confirm that the chief complaint is shortness of breath. Remember that this may be a symptom of conditions affecting systems other than the chest (for example, hypovolaemia due to bleeding). Determine if this is a new problem or an exacerbation of a chronic condition. Ask what precipitated the problem and what, if anything, makes the patient feel more or less breathless. Ask about associated symptoms, such as chest pain, cough and sputum production, palpitations, fever and malaise, and leg pain or swelling. Has the patient been using inhalers or nebulisers more than normal? Have they recently sought other medical assistance?

Enquire about previous similar episodes. If this has occurred before, find out what treatment led to its resolution. Has the patient been hospitalised previously for this condition? What is their general previous medical history? What medications are they currently taking, and why? Are they conforming to their recommended drug regimen, and do they have a good technique when using their inhaler? Is there a family history of respiratory illness or heart disease?

Finally, investigate the patient's social circumstances. Is there evidence of self-neglect? If the patient is not capable of caring for themselves, is there adequate carer support from family, friends, or health and social services? Does the patient smoke? Is there evidence of drug or alcohol abuse that may make the patient susceptible to infection?

Objective examination

Vital signs

The vital signs that should be recorded in a patient with shortness of breath are listed in Box 4.6.

Social context

In addition to the clinical assessment, it is important to consider the patient's ability to care for themselves or whether suitable support mechanisms are available. If these are absent, can they be arranged? Can the patient perform the normal activities of daily living – feeding, washing

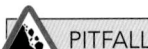 **PITFALL**

Repeated 'practice' attempts to measure maximum PEFR can worsen bronchospasm – limit measurement to best of three forced exhalations

---

BOX 4.6 Vital signs for assessing shortness of breath

- Respiratory rate and effort
- SpO_2
- Peak expiratory flow rate (PEFR)
- Blood pressure
- Orientation and GCS
- Temperature

and using the toilet – either with or without support? The time of day and day of the week may also influence the decision about whether to admit or refer the patient, as this may dictate how quickly a patient could be seen by their own GP or reviewed by the emergency care practitioner.

General examination

Look for signs of the 'unwell' patient (see Chapter 2). A detailed examination of the respiratory system is mandatory for patients with shortness of breath. Remember, however, that myocardial infarction, acute coronary syndromes and congestive cardiac failure can also result in respiratory distress, as may endocrine and neurological problems (for example Kussmaul's and Cheyne–Stokes respiration in hyperglycaemia and raised intra-cranial pressure respectively). If a respiratory problem cannot be readily identified as the cause of the patient's symptoms, undertake an examination of the other systems.

For details of the respiratory examination, refer to Boxes 4.3, 4.5, 4.6 and 4.7 and to Chapter 2. Note if the patient has excessive production of sputum. What colour is this? Yellow, green or brown sputum indicates a chest infection. White frothy sputum, which may also be tinged with pink, suggests pulmonary oedema.

Look at the patient to determine their colour, and for signs of raised jugular venous pressure. Is the patient breathing through pursed lips, or using accessory muscles, perhaps suggesting COPD? Are there signs of CO_2 retention (tremor of the hands, facial flushing, falling conscious level)? Palpate the trachea to check that it is in the midline. Examine the chest and observe chest expansion. Is this the same on both sides? Is there evidence of hyperinflation? Are scars present from surgery? Is there evidence of chest wall deformity?

Feel the chest to confirm equality of movement, and check for chest wall crepitus and surgical emphysema. Is there evidence of chest wall tenderness or pain? Is any pain positional, or worsened on inspiration (as, for example, in pleurisy)? Feel for tactile vocal fremitus (TVF). This is assessed by placing the side of a hand on both sides of the chest in the anterior and posterior upper, middle, and lower zones and asking the patient to say 'ninety-nine'. The resulting low-frequency sounds should normally be palpable, and transmission should be compared for symmetry and differences between the areas assessed.

Listen to the chest. Percuss the anterior and posterior chest wall bilaterally at the top, middle and bottom of the back. Is the percussion note normal, dull or hyper-resonant? Auscultate the chest at the same locations and in the axillae while the patient breathes in and out of an open mouth. Listen for the sounds of bronchial breathing, wheeze or crackles. Listen for vocal resonance and pleural rubs. Vocal resonance is assessed by asking the patient to whisper 'one, two, three' and listening with a stethoscope in the areas described for assessing TVF. Some resonance (although not the words themselves) should normally be

TIP

Elderly patients are likely to have multiple pathologies, so undertake a general systems examination

TIP

Though SOB can result from problems in many systems a useful clue is to note if there is any increase in effort of breathing – this invariably means the problem has a respiratory basis

TIP

If it is uncertain if a percussion note is dull or normal, compare with the result of percussing over the liver (lower ribs on the right); the percussion note will sound dull as the liver is a solid organ

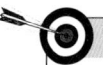 **TIP**

Tactile vocal fremitus and vocal resonance are increased in consolidation and decreased in pleural effusion and pneumothorax

 PITFALL

Do not attempt to examine the upper airway of a child with respiratory distress associated with stridor or drooling. These findings may be indicative of epiglottitis and attempts to examine the mouth and throat may provoke complete airway obstruction.

detected and differences between areas should be noted as described above. Increased sound transmission, demonstrated by clear detection of words spoken by the patient and known as whispering pectoriloquy, is abnormal. Both TVF and vocal resonance are used to assess for the presence of consolidation (increased resonance) or pneumothorax or pleural effusion (decreased resonance).

If the adult patient complains of symptoms of a respiratory tract infection, undertake an ENT examination. Look in the mouth to examine for tonsillar and pharyngeal inflammation, and feel for enlargement of the lymph nodes in the neck.

In all patients with sudden onset of shortness of breath and in the absence of other findings strongly suggestive of a respiratory problem, undertake an examination of the cardiovascular system (see Chapters 2 and 3).

The pertinent features of the respiratory examination are summarised in Box 4.7.

BOX 4.7 Pertinent features of the respiratory examination

General
- Discoloured sputum
- Consider examination of cardiovascular, ENT and other systems

Feel (palpate)
- Chest wall tenderness
- Tactile vocal fremitus
- Percussion note
- Crepitus
- Surgical emphysema

Look (inspect)
- Skin colour
- Jugular venous pressure
- Tracheal deviation
- Breathing through pursed lips
- Use of accessory muscles
- Hand tremor
- Symmetry of chest wall movement
- Hyperinflation or fixed expansion
- Scars from previous surgery
- Chest wall deformity

Listen (auscultate)
- Bronchial breathing, wheeze or crackles
- Vocal resonance
- Pleural rub

Analysis (differential diagnosis)

Diagnosis is often straightforward with a typical history and findings. For example the patient presenting with wheeze and tachypnoea may state that they have asthma. The skill is in determining the *severity* of the condition. Few patients die due to the misdiagnosis of asthma but significant numbers die because professionals or patients underestimate the severity of an attack. Differential diagnosis can also be very difficult, classically in distinguishing between an exacerbation of COPD and cardiogenic pulmonary oedema. This may be made simpler by the use of b-naturetic peptide (BNP) estimations. This has recently been made available as a near-patient test and may become increasingly common in the out-of-hospital setting.

Asthma

The pointers in history and examination in patients with asthma that help to gauge the severity of an attack are summarised in Table 4.1. Patients with severe or life threatening asthma need calm reassurance (even if the healthcare provider is personally anxious), early treatment with beta-2 agonists, oxygen and immediate transfer to hospital. Patients with mild or moderate attacks who respond well to treatment may be suitable for home management with further inhaled beta-2 agonists, oral steroids and early review (Box 4.8 and Table 4.1).[1]

COPD

Exacerbations of COPD are common. These can be triggered by a number of factors but a viral infection is the most frequent. Diagnosis is often simple but it is the assessment of the severity of the condition that needs skill. The main differential diagnosis is of cardiogenic pulmonary oedema (LVF). A pneumothorax is an uncommon reason for a severe sudden exacerbation of COPD. Knowledge of the patient's normal pulmonary function is important. Some patients with COPD have a 'normal' PO_2 that would indicate severe respiratory failure in a normal individual. Signs of exhaustion, inability to expectorate or CO_2 retention are the main worrying features indicating a severe attack.

Oxygen treatment in these patients should be titrated against the SpO_2 (controlled oxygen therapy – see the North-West Oxygen Group guidelines[2]). If the attack is not severe and the patient has adequate home support, then hospital admission may be avoided (Box 4.9).[3]

TABLE 4.1 'Personal best' PEFR values with ranges for estimating severity of acute asthma attack				
If patient's 'personal best' peak flow meter reading is:	Normal variation *above:*	Moderate acute asthma	Severe acute asthma	Life-threatening acute asthma *less than:*
100	80	50 to 80	33 to 50	33
125	100	63 to 100	41 to 63	41
150	120	75 to 120	50 to 75	50
175	140	88 to 140	58 to 88	58
200	160	100 to 160	66 to 100	66
225	180	113 to 180	74 to 113	74
250	200	125 to 200	83 to 125	83
275	220	138 to 220	91 to 138	91
300	240	150 to 240	99 to 150	99
325	260	163 to 260	107 to 163	107
350	280	175 to 280	116 to 175	116
375	300	188 to 300	124 to 188	124
400	320	200 to 320	132 to 200	132
425	340	213 to 340	140 to 213	140
450	360	225 to 360	149 to 225	149
475	380	238 to 380	157 to 238	157
500	400	250 to 400	165 to 250	165
525	420	263 to 420	173 to 263	173
550	440	275 to 440	182 to 275	182
575	460	288 to 460	190 to 288	190
600	480	300 to 480	198 to 300	198

BOX 4.8 Differential diagnosis of asthma

Subjective assessment
History of:
■ Episodic wheezing
■ Nocturnal cough
■ Previous diagnosis
■ Previous episodes requiring intervention additional to maintenance drug therapy
■ Increasing dyspnoea and wheeze
■ Decreasing wheeze in the absence of recovery is a serious finding suggesting grossly inadequate ventilation
■ Precipitating factor, including infection, exercise, exposure to allergen, exposure to cold air
■ Other atopy (e.g. eczema, hay fever)
■ History of previous hospital admission (particularly ICU)/need for ventilation is cause for significant concern, suggesting brittle asthma
 Asthma medications may be evident (inhalers with beta-2 agonists and steroids are usual in adults; nebulisers and oral steroids suggest more significant problems)
 Patient or other household residents may smoke
 Possible limitations in activities of daily living

Objective examination
General findings include wheeze and increasing dyspnoea
 Moderate acute asthma:
■ PEFR >50% normal (see Table 4.1)
■ Normal speech
■ Respirations <25
■ Pulse <110
 Severe acute asthma:
■ PEFR 33–50% of normal (see Table 4.1)
■ Cannot complete sentences
■ Respirations ≧25
■ Pulse ≧110
 Life threatening acute asthma:
■ PEFR <33% of normal (see Table 4.1)
■ SpO_2 <92% on air/<95% on oxygen
■ Silent chest (no wheeze)
■ Cyanosis
■ Feeble respiratory effort
■ Bradycardia or dysrhythmia
■ Hypotension
■ Exhaustion, altered mental status, or falling GCS

BOX 4.9 Differential diagnosis of chronic obstructive pulmonary disease (COPD)

Subjective assessment
History of:
- Previous diagnosis with recent exacerbation
- Increasing wheeze and chest tightness
- Increased sputum production and purulence
- New peripheral oedema
- Episodic deterioration in condition, possibly with hospital admission
- Smoking (common)
- Family history
- Reducing mobility
- Increasing limitations in activities of daily living
- Occupational exposure to dusts, etc.
- Asthma may also be present
  Medications such as beta-2 agonists (inhaler or nebuliser), steroids and antibiotics may be evident
  Chronic bronchitis is defined as a productive cough on most days for 3 months of the year for $\geqq 2$ years

Objective examination
- Hyper-inflated chest
- Increased end-tidal CO_2, decreased SpO_2 and cyanosis (bronchitis and late stage emphysema)
- Normal end-tidal CO_2 and SpO_2 and pink colour (emphysema)
- Increasing dyspnoea on exertion
- Use of accessory muscles of respiration
- Possible productive cough
- Crepitations or wheezes may be present
- Cor pulmonale (right heart failure, e.g. ankle swelling) is a sign of late stage COPD
- Increasing pulse and respiratory rates indicate an exacerbation of COPD
  Note: COPD includes chronic bronchitis (increased airway resistance due to narrowing of the airways) and emphysema (decreased outflow pressure due to loss of elasticity in lung tissues)

Acute cardiogenic pulmonary oedema

The onset is often sudden and severe. The patient is older and usually has a history of ischaemic heart disease although this may be the first indication of heart problems. Acute MI is often a precipitating factor. Severe shortness of breath, white frothy sputum, tachypnoea, tachycardia, pallor and sweating are common. Such patients need to be transported to hospital, sitting upright if possible. Immediate treatment consists of buccal nitrates (providing the blood pressure is not low), oxygen and intravenous opiates (Box 4.10).

BOX 4.10 Differential diagnosis of acute pulmonary oedema
(left ventricular failure/LVF)

Subjective assessment
History of:
- Pre-existing heart disease (undiagnosed chest pain, angina, myocardial infarction, aortic or mitral valve disease, tachyarrhythmias)
- Increasing dyspnoea
- Increasing exercise intolerance
- Rheumatic fever
- Lack of compliance to prescribed medications
- Failure to cope with normal activities of daily living
    Evidence of a wide range of drugs used to treat cardiac conditions may be found, including beta-blockers, calcium channel blockers, ACE inhibitors, nitrates, aspirin, diuretics and anti-arrhythmics

Objective examination
- Severe dyspnoea increased by recumbent positioning. May be worse at night
- Cough producing white frothy sputum, sometimes tinged pink (this may be copious = frank pulmonary oedema)
- Crackles over affected area
- Raised JVP
- Third heart sound (requires practice to differentiate!)
- Mitral murmur (requires practice to differentiate!)
- Possible dysrhythmias
- Hypotension
- Chest pain may be present
- Dependent pitting oedema (generalised heart failure)

Pneumonia

Pyrexia, malaise and purulent sputum suggest a diagnosis of pneumonia. The criteria for home treatment vary from country to country (Box 4.11).[4]

Conditions for exclusion if hospital attendance is not considered appropriate

Box 4.5 lists the key findings that indicate the need for immediate hospital admission in primary survey negative patients. Table 4.2 describes additional findings determined from the secondary survey that will suggest the need for hospital admission. In asthma or COPD, failure to respond to the initial dose of a beta-2 agonist (e.g. nebulised salbutamol) is also an indication for considering hospitalisation, as is a history of a previous near-fatal attack – regardless of the severity of the current episode. All patients with a first episode of pulmonary oedema or an acute exacerbation of a chronic problem should be admitted to hospital for further investigation and treatment.

BOX 4.11 Differential diagnosis of shortness of breath with pyrexia and malaise (pneumonia)

Subjective assessment
History of:
■ Predisposing factors, such as influenza, smoking, suppressed cough reflex (e.g. coma), pulmonary oedema, COPD, alcoholism, immunosuppression, long-term administration of broad spectrum antibiotics, general debility or immobility
■ Contact with person with pneumonia or recent hospital admission (less than 2 weeks previously)
■ Increasing breathlessness
■ Upper/lower respiratory tract infection
■ General malaise
    There may be evidence of failure to cope with normal activities of daily living

Objective examination
■ Increasing dyspnoea
■ Dry cough becoming productive (green purulent sputum)
■ Pyrexia
■ Pleuritic chest pain (worse on inspiration, possibly positional, may be severe)
■ Consolidation:
    – reduced chest wall expansion on side of consolidation
    – dull to percussion over affected area
    – increased TVF and vocal resonance over affected area
■ Crackles over affected area
■ Wheeze
■ Pleuritic rub

Pneumothorax

Spontaneous pneumothorax is most common in tall, thin, fit young men (Table 4.2). It is an uncommon complication of asthma and COPD. There are some rarer causes but these are very uncommon in the community setting. If a pneumothorax is suspected the patient will need to be referred to hospital for an X-ray and further evaluation.

Pulmonary embolism

Half of all patients suffering pulmonary embolism will develop the condition whilst in hospital or long term care. The remainder will have an unknown aetiology or will have been exposed to a known risk factor (see Table 4.2). If a pulmonary embolism is suspected the patient will require urgent transfer to hospital for possible heparinisation or thrombolysis.[5]

TABLE 4.2 Findings from secondary survey suggesting need for hospital admission

Condition	Key findings
Pleural effusion	History of cancer, cardiac failure or renal failure Limited chest expansion on the affected side Dull percussion note over the affected area Reduced breath sounds, TVF and vocal resonance over the affected area Possible crackles in the presence of LVF Possible pleuritic rub (infection) Tracheal shift away from the effusion (late sign)

Pneumothorax (most spontaneous pneumothoraces occur in tall, thin, fit young adults)	Sudden onset of dyspnoea and pleuritic chest pain (early sign)
	Development of tension pneumothorax may be identified by increasing dyspnoea, and:
	    Reduced chest expansion on the affected side
	    Hyper-inflated, fixed chest wall on the affected side
	    Surgical emphysema (rare)
	    Trachea deviated *away* from affected side
	    Chest hyper-resonant to percussion
	    Decreased or absent breath sounds on the affected side
	    Raised JVP
	    Deteriorating cardiovascular status (late sign)

Lung collapse (bronchial obstruction)	Dyspnoea Reduced chest expansion on affected side Tracheal deviation *towards* side of collapse Dull to percussion over non-inflated area Decreased TVF over affected area Breath sounds absent or decreased over affected area; increased bronchial breathing elsewhere

Pulmonary embolism (PE)	Clinical features compatible with PE:
	    (a) Dyspnoea *and/or*
	    (b) Tachypnoea (> 20 breaths per minute) *and*
	    (c) Haemoptysis *and/or*
	    (d) Pleuritic chest pain
	Major risk factors for PE:
	    (a) Major abdominal or pelvic surgery
	    (b) Hip or knee replacement
	    (c) Post-operative intensive care
	    (d) Late pregnancy
	    (e) Caesarean section
	    (f) Puerperium
	    (g) Lower limb fracture
	    (h) Varicose veins
	    (i) Abdominal, pelvic, or metastatic malignancy
	    (j) Reduced mobility due to hospitalisation or institutional care
	    (k) Previous history of venous thromboembolism
	In the absence of another reasonable clinical explanation for the signs and symptoms:
	    If (a), (b) and (c) are all confirmed the likelihood of PE is high;
	    If (a) and (b) *or* (c) are present the likelihood of PE is intermediate;
	    If (a) is present but (b) *and* (c) are both absent the likelihood of PE is low, especially in cases of pleuritic chest pain or haemoptysis *not* accompanied by breathlessness

Treatment and disposal (plan)

The initial out-of-hospital treatment of each of the four key conditions is given in Table 4.3 and Boxes 4.12 to 4.14. Interventions recommended in the JRCALC guidelines for paramedic use are asterisked.[6]

TABLE 4.3 Treatment of asthma[2]		
Moderate acute asthma	Severe acute asthma (or no response to treatment in moderate asthma)	Life threatening acute asthma
Protect and maintain airway as necessary	Oxygen via non-rebreathing mask*	Oxygen via non-rebreathing mask*
Position for comfort (usually sitting upright)	Give salbutamol 5 mg nebuliser*	Give salbutamol 5 mg nebuliser mixed with ipratropium 0.5 mg*
Salbutamol 5 mg via oxygen driven nebuliser	Administer prednisolone 40–50 mg orally or hydrocortisone 100 mg IV*	Commence transportation to hospital
If PEFR >50–75% of normal, give prednisolone 40–50 mg orally	If no response, give salbutamol 5 mg nebuliser mixed with ipratropium 0.5 mg*	Administer prednisolone 40–50 mg orally or hydrocortisone 200 mg IV*
Treat and leave if patient responds to treatment	Give continuous salbutamol 5 mg nebulisers until symptoms are controlled	Give continuous salbutamol 5 mg nebulisers until symptoms are controlled
Arrange re-assessment, possibly by telephone, at a suitable time	*Consider* treat and leave if patient fully responds to treatment and has adequate carer support	Consider intravenous crystalloids in the presence of dehydration to limit mucous plugging
Consider referring to GP or specialist nurse for delayed follow-up if patient requires further support or review of treatment	If discharged, arrange re-assessment, possibly by telephone, at a suitable time	Refer to GP for immediate appointment

PITFALL

Tension pneumothorax is a rare complication of asthma and COPD. Monitor for its signs and perform needle thoracocentesis (decompression) if these are present

 TIP

Check the inhaler technique of patients left at home[7]

 PITFALL

Rule out acute MI: if present consider opiates, nitrates, aspirin, heparin and thrombolysis according to relevant guidelines

---

BOX 4.12 Treatment of COPD[3]

- Protect and maintain airway as necessary*
- Position for comfort (usually sitting upright)*
- Salbutamol 5 mg via nebuliser*
- Ipratropium 0.5 mg via nebuliser (may be mixed with salbutamol)
- Re-assess: if patient's condition returns to their normal state, consider managing at home:
    - confirm appropriate technique when using inhalers
    - consider increasing dose of bronchodilator
    - consider oral steroids if:
    – previous documented response to steroid therapy
    – dyspnoea is increasing despite prior increase in bronchodilator dose
- Consider antibiotics if two or more of the following are present:
    - increasing dyspnoea
    - increasing sputum volume
    - development of purulent sputum
- Refer to GP for appointment for re-assessment within 24 hours
    If no response to initial nebuliser, transport to hospital. On route:
- Repeat salbutamol 5 mg nebuliser at 5 min intervals until symptoms are controlled*
- Administer oxygen at 24–28% via Venturi mask initially
- Monitor SpO_2 and adjust oxygen concentration to maintain at 'usual' level for patient or at 90–92% if unknown (see North West Oxygen Group guidelines[2])
- Consider supporting ventilation if SpO_2 cannot be maintained, patient becomes exhausted or respiratory rate or effort declines inappropriate

---

BOX 4.13 Treatment of acute pulmonary oedema

All patients with an acute exacerbation of pulmonary oedema require hospitalisation
- Protect and maintain airway as necessary*
- Position for comfort (usually sitting upright)*
- Oxygen via non-rebreathing mask*
- Use Continuous Positive Airway Pressure ventilation (CPAP) if available; otherwise consider assisting ventilations with BVM if respiratory failure evident
- 400 µg glyceryl trinitrate spray if systolic BP >90 mmHg*
- Consider recording 12-lead ECG
- Commence transportation to hospital*
- Consider second dose of GTN if SBP >90 mmHg*
- Give furosemide 40 mg IV*
- Give morphine 5–20 mg IV (monitor respirations and assist ventilation if respiratory depression becomes evident)
- Consider repeating furosemide 40 mg IV at 10-minute intervals to a maximum dose of 120 mg*
- Consider salbutamol 5 mg via nebuliser in the presence of wheeze*
- Consider further GTN 400 µg if SBP >90 mmHg

BOX 4.14 Treatment of pneumonia[4]

If no evidence of respiratory failure or severe respiratory distress, and the patient has adequate carer support and can manage normal daily activities of living (see Chapter 3):
- position for comfort (usually sitting upright)
- antibiotic therapy
- refer to GP for appointment for follow-up within 24 hours
  In the absence of adequate carer support and if unable to manage daily tasks of living, or if tachycardia, tachypnoea or chest pain are present:
- consider hospital admission
- oxygen via non-rebreathing mask if required to maintain SpO_2 above 95%
- consider intravenous crystalloids in the presence of dehydration

---

Disposition flow chart

Figure 4.2 describes the decision-making process for patient disposition.

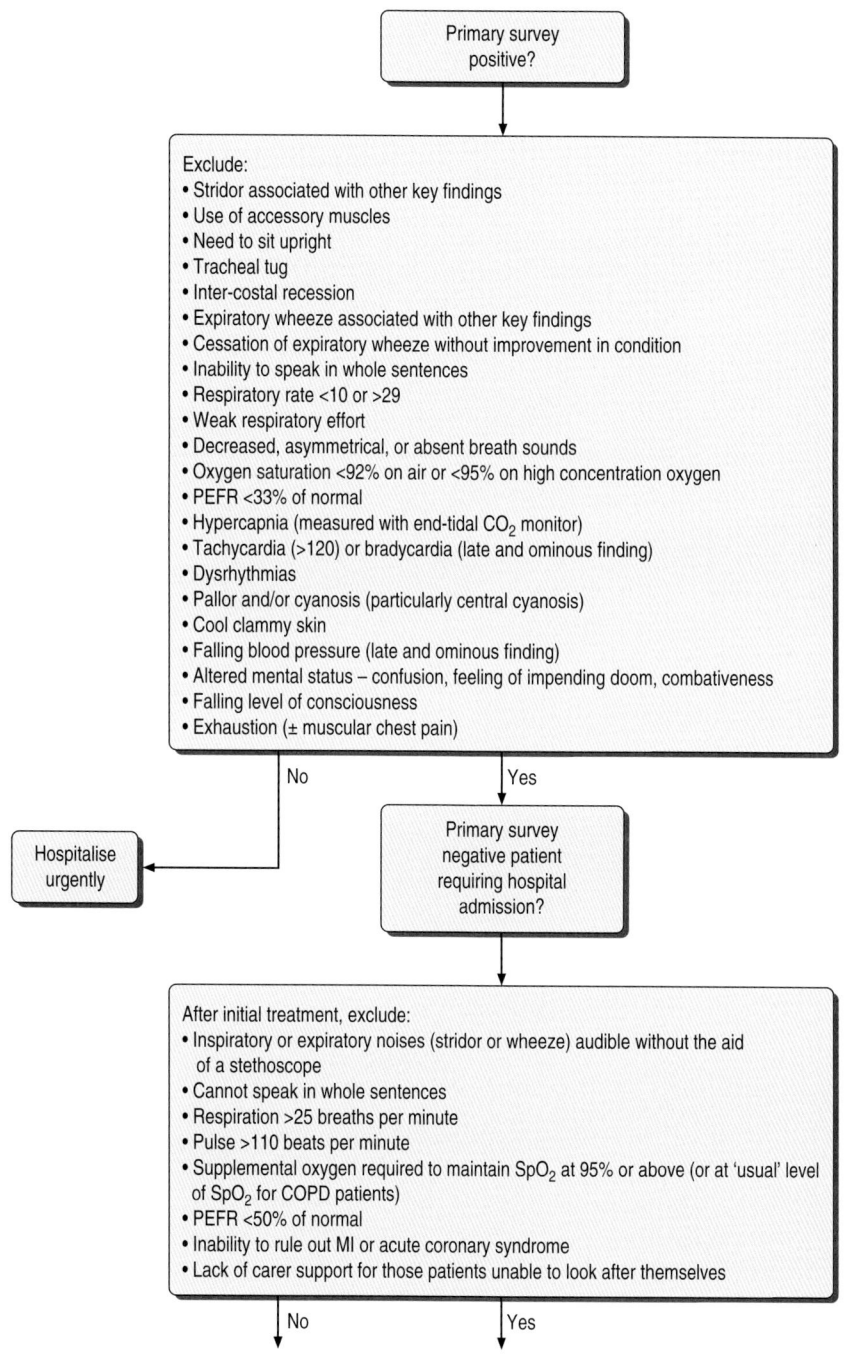

Primary survey
positive?

Exclude:
• Stridor associated with other key findings
• Use of accessory muscles
• Need to sit upright
• Tracheal tug
• Inter-costal recession
• Expiratory wheeze associated with other key findings
• Cessation of expiratory wheeze without improvement in condition
• Inability to speak in whole sentences
• Respiratory rate <10 or >29
• Weak respiratory effort
• Decreased, asymmetrical, or absent breath sounds
• Oxygen saturation <92% on air or <95% on high concentration oxygen
• PEFR <33% of normal
• Hypercapnia (measured with end-tidal CO_2 monitor)
• Tachycardia (>120) or bradycardia (late and ominous finding)
• Dysrhythmias
• Pallor and/or cyanosis (particularly central cyanosis)
• Cool clammy skin
• Falling blood pressure (late and ominous finding)
• Altered mental status – confusion, feeling of impending doom, combativeness
• Falling level of consciousness
• Exhaustion (± muscular chest pain)

No   Yes

Hospitalise urgently

Primary survey
negative patient
requiring hospital
admission?

After initial treatment, exclude:
• Inspiratory or expiratory noises (stridor or wheeze) audible without the aid
  of a stethoscope
• Cannot speak in whole sentences
• Respiration >25 breaths per minute
• Pulse >110 beats per minute
• Supplemental oxygen required to maintain SpO_2 at 95% or above (or at 'usual' level
  of SpO_2 for COPD patients)
• PEFR <50% of normal
• Inability to rule out MI or acute coronary syndrome
• Lack of carer support for those patients unable to look after themselves

No   Yes

Fig. 4.2 Disposition flow chart (shortness of breath)

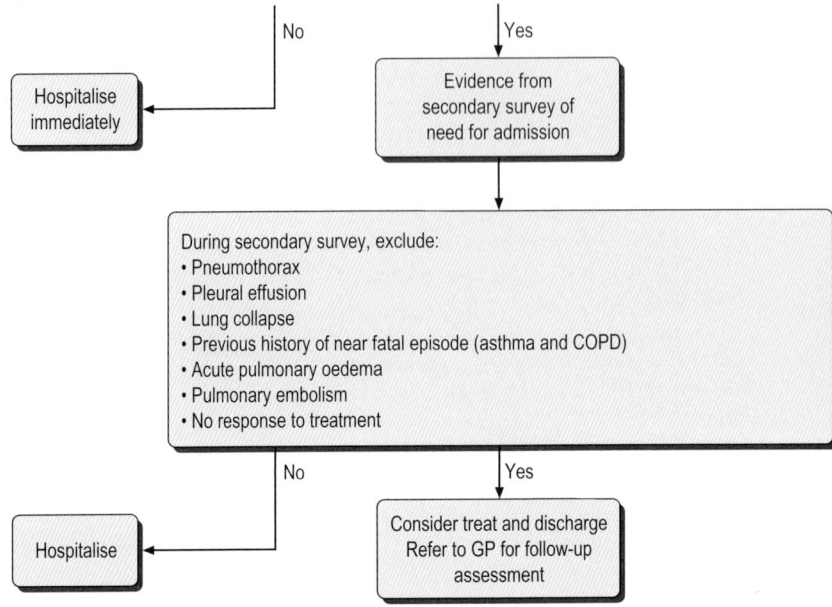

Fig. 4.2—Cont'd   Disposition flow chart (shortness of breath)

Follow-up

Patients with an acute exacerbation of the conditions discussed in this paper but not requiring hospital admission should be advised to request further assistance if their condition deteriorates once the carer has left. Reassessment of the need for hospital admission is then mandatory.

All patients provided with home care should be referred for an appointment with their General Practitioner within a suitable time frame for further assessment. This will include consideration of the patient's ongoing condition, their ability to use inhalers correctly, measurement of their respiratory function (FEV1), and life style management advice (e.g. smoking cessation, weight control, exercise).

Acknowledgements

Thanks to Jim Wardrope, Peter Driscoll and Colville Laird whose feedback resulted in valuable improvements to earlier drafts of this chapter.

References

1 BTS/SIGN 2003 The BTS/SIGN British guideline on the management of asthma. Thorax 58(suppl 1): i1–i94
2 Murphy R, Mackway-Jones K, Sammy I, et al 2001 Emergency oxygen therapy for the breathless patient. Guidelines prepared by North West Oxygen Group. J Accid Emerg Med 18:420–423
3 The British Thoracic Society Standards of Care Committee 1997 Guidelines on the Management of COPD. Thorax 52 (suppl 5): S1–S28
4 The British Thoracic Society 2001 Guidelines for the management of community acquired pneumonia in adults. Thorax 56 (suppl 4): iv1–iv64
5 The British Thoracic Society Standards of Care Committee Pulmonary Embolism Guideline Development Group 2003 BTS guidelines for the management of suspected acute pulmonary embolism, 2003. Thorax 58:470–484
6 Joint Royal Colleges Ambulance Liaison Committee 2002 Pre-hospital Guidelines version 2.1. JRCALC/Ambulance Service Association, London
7 National asthma campaign 2004 How to use your inhaler. Available online: http://www.asthma.org.uk/using_your.html (5 Mar 2007)

Further reading

Marsh J 1999 Respiratory examination. In: Marsh J. Crash course. History and examination. Mosby International, London

O'Conner D J, Jones B G 2002 Pathology of the respiratory system. In: O'Conner D J, JonesB G. Crash course. Pathology, 2nd edn. Mosby International, London

The British Thoracic Society website contains extensive information about respiratory illness and relevant guidelines. Available online: http://www. brit-thoracic.org.uk (5 Mar 2007)

Wardle T 1999 Respiratory emergencies. In: Greaves I, Porter K (eds) Pre-hospital medicine. The principles and practice of immediate care. Arnold, London

The ill child – assessment and identification of primary survey positive children

Introduction

Sick children present particular challenges to the pre-hospital practitioner. The anatomy of children is different to that of adults, and this can result in differences in the presentation and severity of a range of conditions. Paediatric physiology also differs from that of adults, and although this means children often compensate very well for significant clinical illness it also carries the risk that a severe problem will be overlooked or underestimated. When compensatory mechanisms fail in children, they often do so rapidly, catastrophically and irreversibly. The index of suspicion of the pre-hospital practitioner must therefore be higher than for an adult when assessing the ill child, and the threshold for hospital admission will consequently be lower than for an adult patient with similar findings. The emphasis should be on detecting and treating the seriously ill child at an early stage to prevent deterioration rather than to attempting to cope with a decompensated, critically ill child.

The paediatric section of this text is divided into two chapters. The objectives of this first chapter are outlined in Box 5.1.

Whilst this chapter concentrates on identifying or ruling out potentially time critical problems, it should be remembered that many children have problems that are not immediately life threatening. Common illnesses affecting children are covered in Chapter 6.

BOX 5.1 Chapter objectives

- To describe the anatomical and physiological differences between children and adults
- To describe the range of normal behaviours in children of different ages
- To discuss approaches to assessing children to minimise the effects of distress
- To identify the findings associated with primary survey positive patients
- To differentiate between compensating and decompensating primary survey positive patients
- To discuss where treatment should be initiated in primary survey positive patients
- To identify consent issues in caring for children
- To discuss child protection issues

Significant anatomical and physiological differences between children and adults

Airway

In infants (aged 0–1 years) and children (aged 1–8 years) the head is proportionately larger and the neck shorter than in adults. This can lead to neck flexion in the recumbent baby or child, precipitating airway obstruction. The trachea is also more malleable, and this coupled with the large tongue can result in airway obstruction if the head is over-extended when attempting to open the airway by positioning, particularly in infants. Milk teeth may be loose, and the smaller size of the mouth increases the risk of dislodgment or tissue damage. Compressing the surface of the skin below the lower jaw in an attempt to open the airway can result in the tongue being displaced and worsening obstruction. Infants less than 6 months old are obligate nasal breathers. The epiglottis is horseshoe shaped and the larynx higher and more anterior, the tracheal rings are soft and not fully formed, and the cricoid cartilage is the narrowest part of the upper airway. All have implications for airway management and the consequences of related illnesses.

Breathing

The total surface area of the lungs and the number of small airways is limited in infants and children and small diameters throughout the respiratory system increase the risk of obstruction. Infants have ribs that lie more horizontally and therefore rely predominantly on the diaphragm for breathing. They are more prone to muscle fatigue and therefore respiratory failure. Increased metabolic rate and oxygen consumption contribute to higher respiratory rates than in adults (Table 5.1).

TABLE 5.1 Vital signs in children			
Age (years)	Breaths per minute	Heart rate	Systolic BP
<1	30–40	110–160	70–90
1–5	25–30	95–140	80–100
5–12	20–25	80–120	90–110
>12	15–20	60–100	100–120

Circulation

Infants and children have a relatively small stroke volume but a higher cardiac output than in adults, facilitated by higher heart rates (Table 5.1). Stroke volume increases with age as heart rate falls, but until the age of two the ability of the child to increase stroke volume is limited. Systemic vascular resistance is lower in infants and children, evidenced by lower systolic blood pressure (Table 5.1). The circulating volume to body weight ratio of children is higher than adults at 80–100 ml/kg (decreasing with age) but the total circulating volume is low. A comparatively small amount of fluid loss can therefore have significant clinical effects.

Other considerations

The surface area of children and infants is high, and this results in rapid heat loss and, coupled with the immature temperature regulation systems of infants, presents an increased risk of hypothermia. Glycogen stores in the liver are limited and hypoglycaemia can be present in any child that has been too ill to feed or subjected to high metabolic demands due to illness or trauma.

Range of normal development in children, and assessment strategies

Infants

The developmental milestones of infants are outlined in Table 5.2. Remember, there may be wide variation in the age of attaining these milestones.

When assessing an infant, the caregiver can be asked to hold the child and get down to 'baby level'. It is a good idea to say the child's name,

TABLE 5.2 Developmental milestones in infants

Age (months)	Activity
< 2	Predominantly sleeping or eating Unable to differentiate between strangers and carers/family
2–6	Spends more time awake Starting to make eye contact May follow movement of toys/lights with eyes May turn head towards sounds Starts to vocalise sounds Active extremity movements May recognise caregivers
7–12	Sits unsupported Reaches for objects and puts them in mouth Recognises caregivers and afraid of separation from them; afraid of strangers

speak softly and avoid sudden movements. The examination may be commenced by simply observing the child, and then 'hands on' examination can begin starting with the least upsetting steps. It is wise to adjust the order of the examination according to the child's behaviour – for example, listening to breath sounds and counting the respiratory rate when the child is calm and certainly before doing anything that may be painful or distressing. Your hands and any instruments should be warm, and clothing should be removed only one item at a time to maintain body warmth and reduce fear.

Children

The developmental milestones for children aged 1–12 are outlined in Table 5.3.

The child can be observed from a distance initially whilst the history is being taken, and then approached slowly, preferably avoiding physical contact until the child is familiar with you. Children should remain with caregivers, and sit on their lap if they wish to do so. Young children respond to praise – admiring clothes or a favourite toy and recognising good behaviour are effective ways to win them over. They may

TABLE 5.3 Range of normal behaviours in children aged 1 to 12 years	
Age (years)	Activity
1–2	Initially crawling and walking supported by furniture, then walking and running Feed themselves Plays with toys Starting to communicate with increasing vocabulary; will understand more than they can vocalise Independent and opinionated: cannot be reasoned with Curious but with no sense of danger Frightened of strangers
2–5	Illogical thinkers (by adult standards) May misinterpret what is said to them Fearful of being left alone, loss of control, and being unwell Limited attention span
5–12	Talkative Understand the relationship between cause and effect Pleased to learn new skills Older children may understand simple explanations about how their bodies work and their illness Fearful about separation from parents, loss of control, pain and disability May be unable to express their thoughts Desire to 'fit in' with peers

be soothed by being allowed to play with their own toys or by being allowed to hold instruments such as a stethoscope. The caregiver can assist with the assessment, by removing clothes or holding an oxygen mask. Use of very simple words and toys can facilitate explanations to the child. Critical parts of the assessment can be undertaken whenever the child is at their most calm: consider examining from toes to head. A limited element of control can be given to the child, asking which part the child would like you to examine first. Do not lie to children and, in particular, never tell them something will not hurt if it will!

School-age children should be addressed directly. Using simple terms, an explanation of what you are going to do, what you think is wrong, and what is going to happen can be given, but the amount of information provided should be limited. Interventions should be explained immediately before undertaking them but negotiation about whether or not to perform necessary procedures is not usually rewarding in young children. Praise for co-operation is a good idea. Children are modest and this should be borne in mind by limiting the removal of clothing and the presence of non-caregivers.

Adolescents

Adolescents may indulge in risk-taking behaviours and have a strong desire to 'fit in' with their peers. They may start to depend more on their friends for social support than their parents and will begin to exert their independence. They will be particularly modest about their bodies and how others see them, and will fear disfigurement. Mood swings are common and although it may be possible to rationalise with teenagers, illness can result in a return to more immature developmental levels of behaviour.

When assessing adolescents their permission should be sought, rather than that of the caregivers, and an explanation given of what you are doing and why. Questions should be encouraged and privacy and confidentiality respected. It is important to be non-judgemental. If necessary, seek the support of the teenager's friends in persuading them to accept treatment.

Children with special learning needs

Children with special learning needs may have a behavioural range that is equivalent to a child younger than their true age in years. Parents or carers will be able to advise what is normal for the child, and you should use the approach appropriate for the child's mental rather than actual age. However, it is important to remember that children with a *physical* disability will often have a normal mental age for their years and they should be communicated with accordingly.

Primary survey positive patients

Primary survey positive children fall into one of two groups. Those who are seriously ill but are currently compensating require immediate transportation to definitive care to prevent further deterioration. Pre-hospital treatment for this group of patients should be given en route: treatment that cannot be practically administered by a single practitioner in the back of a moving ambulance should be postponed until arrival at hospital, unless the patient decompensates prior to arrival. Those that are seriously ill but are no longer able to compensate will require some life-saving interventions 'on-scene' before transportation to hospital but this should be strictly limited to that which will allow delivery of a live child to the emergency department.

Recognition

The main features of the primary survey for children are described in Box 5.2.

 PITFALL

Cessation of wheeze in a child with severe asthma may be misinterpreted as an improvement in the patient's condition

 TIP

Measure capillary refill time centrally, on the forehead or sternum

 TIP

Floppiness of new onset should be assumed to indicate serious illness until proven otherwise

 TIP

Remember: ABCDEFG = ABCs plus Don't Ever Forget the Glucose

 PITFALL

Peripheral cyanosis is normal in babies up to approx. 3 months

---

BOX 5.2 Main features of paediatric primary survey

Airway
- Is the airway noisy (snoring, stridor, wheeze, grunting, muffled or hoarse speech)?

Work of breathing
- Will the child lie flat? Are they in the tripod or 'sniffing' position?
- Are accessory muscles being used (head bobbing in infants)? Or is there minimal movement of the chest wall?
- Is there sternal, supra-clavicular, sub-sternal or intercostal recession present?
- Is nasal flaring present?
- Is the respiratory rate fast, slow or normal?
- Is cyanosis present?
- Is there a very recent history of wheezing that has now stopped?
- Is air movement audible on auscultation?
- What is the SpO_2?

Circulation
- Is skin colour normal, or is it pale or mottled?
- Is there an increased respiratory rate without increased work of breathing?
- What is the temperature of the skin? Is it cool peripherally but warm centrally?
- Is the pulse rate fast, slow or normal?
- Is the pulse volume weak or strong?
- Is the capillary refill time normal or prolonged?

Disability
- What is the AVPU score? (Alert, response to Verbal stimuli, response to Pain, Unresponsive)
- Is the child mobile? Do they run away? Or is there limited movement with poor muscle tone?
- Do they interact with carers or toys or are they disinterested or unresponsive?
- If they are crying or speaking, is this strong or weak?
- If crying, can they be consoled?
- Do they fix their gaze on responders or carers, or do they have a 'glazed' appearance?
- Is the child's behaviour normal for their developmental age?
- Is the child fitting?
- Is the child stiff or floppy?

Exposure
- Is there evidence of pyrexia?
- Is there a non-blanching rash present?
- What is the blood glucose level?

Decompensating primary survey positive patients

Table 5.4 describes the significant findings and pre-transportation treatment for children who are primary survey positive and decompensating. To minimise distress, parents should be encouraged to hold small children who remain alert.

Once life-saving interventions have been initiated, the child should be moved to the ambulance and transported immediately, continuing treatment en route as described in Table 5.5.

TABLE 5.4 Recognition and pre-transportation treatment of the decompensating primary survey positive patient

Problem	Findings	Pre-transportation treatment
Respiratory failure	Noisy upper airway becoming quiet without improvement in condition	Secure airway using the most simple manoeuvre if possible: use advanced interventions (e.g. intubation) only if simple manoeuvres fail
	Very rapid and shallow or slow weak respirations	Give high concentration oxygen via non-rebreathing mask
	Decreasing evidence of increased work of breathing due to exhaustion	Consider assisting ventilation with bag valve mask if respiratory rate is very fast or slow
	Significantly decreased air entry on auscultation	In the presence of wheeze consider nebulisation with beta-2 agonist and anti-cholinergic (e.g. salbutamol and ipratropium)
	Limited chest expansion	Consider nebulised epinephrine in the presence of suspected croup (1 ml of 1:1000 once only)
	Loss of wheeze without improvement in condition	Decompress tension pneumothorax
	SpO_2 less than 90% on high concentration oxygen	Consider transmucosal glucose (Hypostop) or intravenous/intraosseous 10% dextrose 5ml/kg
	Cyanosis	
	Reduced AVPU score	
	Flaccid or increased muscle tone	
	No interaction with carers or responders	
	Glazed, unfocused gaze	
	Abnormal, weak or absent cry	
	Hypoglycaemia	
Circulatory failure	Increased respiratory rate in the absence of increased work of breathing	Secure airway using simple manoeuvres if possible: use advanced interventions (e.g. intubation) only if simple manoeuvres fail
	Central pallor, mottling or cyanosis	Give high concentration oxygen via non-rebreathing mask
	Cool skin centrally	Consider intravenous/intraosseous fluid challenge of 5 ml/kg (repeat up to 20 ml/kg)
	Bradycardia or falling heart rate in the absence of improvement in condition	Consider intravenous/intraosseous 10% dextrose 5 ml/kg

(Continued)

TABLE 5.4 Recognition and pre-transportation treatment of the decompensating primary survey positive patient—Cont'd

Problem	Findings	Pre-transportation treatment
	Central capillary refill time >5 seconds or absent Reduced AVPU score Flaccid muscle tone No interaction with carers or responders Glazed, unfocused gaze Weak or absent cry Non-blanching rash in an ill child	Consider benzylpenicillin IV or IM
Central nervous system failure	Reduced AVPU score	Consider the presence of undiagnosed respiratory or circulatory failure and treat accordingly. Otherwise:
	Flaccid muscle tone	Secure airway using simple manoeuvres if possible: use advanced interventions (e.g. intubation) only if simple manoeuvres fail
	No interaction with carers or responders	Give high concentration oxygen via non-rebreathing mask
	Glazed, unfocused gaze	Consider assisting ventilation with bag valve mask if respiratory rate is very fast or slow
	Weak or absent cry	Consider rectal diazepam (0–1 year 2.5 mg, 1–3 years 5 mg, 4–12 years 10 mg) or IV diazepam 250–400 µg/kg, but do not delay to obtain IV access
	Continuous fits, or failure to regain consciousness between fits	Consider transmucosal glucose (Hypostop) or intravenous/intraosseous 10% dextrose 5 ml/kg
	Hypoglycaemia	

TABLE 5.5 Findings associated with compensating primary survey positive patients and en route treatment

Problem	Findings	Treatment en route to hospital
Respiratory distress	Noisy upper airway (snoring, stridor, muffled or hoarse speech)	Secure airway using simple manoeuvres if possible: use advanced interventions (e.g. intubation) only if simple manoeuvres fail
	Grunting	Give high concentration oxygen via non-rebreathing mask
	Increased respiratory rate	Consider nebulised budesonide in the presence of suspected croup (2 mg once only) or oral steroids (dexamethasone syrup 0.15 mg/kg)

TABLE 5.5 Findings associated with compensating primary survey positive patients and en route treatment—Cont'd

Problem	Findings	Treatment en route to hospital
	Refuses to lie flat, or adopts tripod or sniffing position	In the presence of wheeze consider nebulisation with beta-2 agonist and anti-cholinergic (e.g. salbutamol and ipratropium)
	Use of accessory muscles (head bobbing in infants) Sternal, sub-sternal, supra-clavicular or intercostal recession present Nasal flaring Increased or asymmetrical chest expansion Wheezing SpO$_2$ less than 94% on room air Pallor or peripheral cyanosis Normal AVPU score Good muscle tone; may be playing with toys Interacts with carers or responders Focused gaze Strong cry	
Compensated shock	Increased respiratory rate in the absence of increased work of breathing	Secure airway using simple manoeuvres if appropriate: use advanced interventions (e.g. intubation) only if simple manoeuvres fail
	Peripheral pallor, mottling or cyanosis	Give high concentration oxygen via non-rebreathing mask
	Cool skin peripherally, warm centrally	Consider intravenous fluids 20 ml/kg (unless uncontrolled bleeding in which case use 5 ml/kg aliquots)
	Prolonged capillary refill >2 seconds centrally Increased heart rate Normal AVPU score Good muscle tone; may be playing with toys Interacts with carers or responders Focused gaze Strong cry	

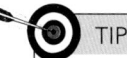 TIP

Remember to pre-alert the receiving hospital of your estimated time of arrival and the child's age and condition

PITFALL

In cases of suspected epiglottitis or severe croup in a spontaneously breathing child withhold all interventions. Never attempt to examine the airway, use airway adjuncts, to remove the child from their carer, or to do anything that may increase distress. Administration of oxygen should be attempted but keep the tubing/mask at a distance that avoids upsetting the child

 TIP

In cases of suspected epiglottitis or severe croup with respiratory arrest initially attempt ventilation with a pocket mask with oxygen or bag–valve–mask. If this is impossible and laryngoscopy and intubation are required but the glottis is obscured by swollen tissue, ask an assistant to press down on the chest and hold it in compression. If a bubble appears, attempt to pass an endotracheal tube through it. If this fails, perform needle cricothyroidotomy

 TIP

Patients with an altered level of consciousness or with limited interaction with carers in the presence or absence of abnormal respiratory or circulatory signs should be considered to be *decompensating*

Compensating primary survey positive children

Seriously ill but compensating children will have signs of either shock or respiratory distress but will have a relatively normal appearance and level of consciousness. Transportation to hospital should be commenced immediately for such patients and whatever appropriate treatment from Table 5.4 that is practical to initiate in a moving ambulance provided en route. Parents should be encouraged to hold small children to minimise distress.

The findings associated with compensating primary survey positive patients and recommendations for en route treatment are described in Table 5.5.

Primary survey negative children with need for early hospital attendance

Primary survey negative patients with the findings listed in Box 5.3 usually require hospital assessment and may need admission.

Parents may have requested the assistance of healthcare providers after using the Baby Check scoring system.[1] This uses a simple 19-point check list to help parents assess the severity of illness in babies up to 6 months old, and to determine the need for medical assessment.

BOX 5.3 Diagnostic criteria for primary survey negative patients requiring hospital admission

Some conditions suggesting need for early hospital review in primary survey negative patients:
- Sudden onset of noisy upper airway in the absence of respiratory distress or altered mentation
- Suspected foreign body inhalation
- History of apnoeic episode (child well on arrival of pre-hospital practitioner)
- Asthma refractory to bronchodilators
- Inability to feed
- Non-blanching rash in an otherwise well child
- First fit of any cause, including febrile convulsions
- Unexpected increase in number of fits in a child prone to convulsions
- More than one fit in a 24-hour period in a febrile child
- Pyrexia >38.5°C in a child under 6 months
- Deliberate overdose or poisoning
- Deliberate self-harm
- Uncontrolled pain
- Suspected child abuse

Consent to treatment

Children (i.e. patients under the age of 18) can be classified into three groups with respect to legal considerations regarding consent for treatment, or its refusal. It is good clinical practice to always attempt to obtain consent from any child requiring treatment, but the following underpinning principles should be adhered to. The doctrine of necessity may be applied if life saving treatment is required for a child or young person in any of these groups and consent cannot be obtained in a timely manner in the required way.

Young person over the age of 16

Young people over the age of 16 should normally be treated as competent adults. Informed consent to treatment should be sought from the patient. Adults with parental responsibility may *not* refuse treatment on behalf of the minor if the young person has consented to it. Adults with parental responsibility may, however, over-ride the decision of a minor to *refuse* life-saving treatment, as may a court of law. If both a young person and those with parental responsibility refuse life-saving treatment this can be over-ridden by a court of law or, in an emergency, health professionals. 'Parental responsibility' is defined in Box 5.4.

> **BOX 5.4 Parental responsibility**
>
> Parental responsibility is given to the following adults by the Children's Act 1989:
> - Both parents if married at any time since the child's conception
> - The mother alone if the child is illegitimate, unless the father has obtained agreement of the mother or a court order
> - A local authority if the child is in care or under a care order
> - An appointed guardian
> - Those with a residence order
> - Adoptive parents
> - Those with an Emergency Protection Order (usually a local authority)

In the event that a young person over the age of 16 does not have competence to understand the proposal regarding treatment, consent may be obtained from those with responsibility or, if this is not immediately available, the doctrine of necessity can be applied.

Child or young person under the age of 16 who is 'Gillick aware' ('Gillick competent')

'Gillick awareness' is defined as the child or young person having achieved sufficient understanding and intelligence to fully understand the treatment that is being suggested. The principles described for minors over the age of 16 should be applied to patients *under* 16 who are 'Gillick aware'. The law assumes that a child under the age of 16 refusing life-saving treatment is unlikely to be Gillick aware and is not, therefore, competent to decline treatment.

Child or young person under the age of 16 who is *not* 'Gillick aware'

If possible, obtain informed consent to treatment from an adult with parental responsibility (see Box 5.4) as well as the child. If such an adult is not immediately available and treatment cannot be delayed, the legal doctrine of necessity may be invoked if the treatment is necessary to save life, ensure improvement, or prevent deterioration in health. The doctrine of necessity can only apply if the treatment provided is in accordance with normal current medical practice and is restricted to that required until parental consent can be obtained.

If those with parental responsibility refuse treatment, a court order should be sought. If this is not feasible because treatment is life-saving and cannot be delayed, the practitioner should discuss the need for the treatment in detail and document this in the presence of a witness.

If possible, a colleague should provide a supporting written recommendation that the treatment is necessary and appropriate, and a defence union contacted.

Child protection

Healthcare providers have a duty of care to be alert to the signs of possible child abuse. This may occur in the form of neglect, physical injury, or sexual or emotional abuse, and may be perpetrated by other children as well as adults.

Identifying potential abuse

A range of pointers to child abuse may be present. Behavioural pointers may be the first alerting sign – either in the carer or child. A variety of behaviours may be manifest – in the carer, delay in seeking help, changing or vague stories as to how an injury occurred, indifference or overprotection should all alert the healthcare professional to assess the situation further. The child may disclose abuse directly (not very common), or may appear fearful or indifferent towards the carer. Abuse may manifest itself as poor behaviour in school, bedwetting or failure to thrive. In short, any unusual pattern of behaviour in either the carer or child should alert the professional to the possibility that the child may be being abused.

The child may tell health professionals that they have been abused, but more often an abnormal pattern of behaviour will suggest a problem. The child may not seek comfort from their parent or carer, and may be unusually willing to go to a previously unknown health worker. They may appear withdrawn or frightened – 'frozen watchfulness' may indicate repetitive abuse. A knowledge of basic developmental milestones can be very useful – for example if a 2-month-old baby is said to have crawled to the edge of the bed and then fallen off it, it is very unlikely to be true.

Physical signs of abuse can include multiple injuries with different stages of healing, such as bruises of different coloration or fractures of different ages. Long bone or rib fractures in young children with limited mobility may suggest the suspicion of violence, as can spinal and head injuries. Soft tissue injuries associated with abuse include cigarette burns or immersion scalds of hands or feet, and imprints of hands, belts or other objects and human bite marks.

Sexual abuse should be considered in the presence of sexual knowledge unusual for the age of the child, unexplained pregnancy, sexually transmitted disease, or injuries to the perineum or sexual organs.

Taking action

All healthcare professionals have a duty of care to report any child that might be at risk from abuse to the appropriate authorities and should be familiar with their organisation's procedures for child welfare and protection. However, in the event that child abuse is suspected, it is not the role of healthcare workers to undertake an investigation. In particular, children should not be asked leading questions as this may prejudice any future criminal enquiry. Concerns should be referred to Social Services without delay or, in the event that immediate action is required, to the police. Child protection policies should document how to make contact with the appropriate organisations outside of normal working hours. Verbal notifications must be followed-up with a written report, and all findings and concerns should be documented in the patient record in detail. It is a good idea to ensure that a referral not requiring immediate action is acknowledged in writing: if it is not, this should be followed up with the relevant agency.

If a child reports abuse, they should be spoken to in a language appropriate to their age. However, it is important not to promise that information will not be disclosed to the appropriate agencies.

In the event that there are concerns that a child is at immediate risk of further harm, parents or carers should be persuaded if possible that hospital admission is appropriate. Practitioners should never behave in a judgemental manner towards parents or reveal their suspicions to them. If a child is perceived to be in immediate danger and it is not possible to remove them to hospital, the police should be contacted immediately. They have the power to legally remove the child to safety.

Acknowledgements

Thanks to Jim Wardrope, Peter Driscoll and Colville Laird whose feedback resulted in improvements to earlier drafts of this paper.

Reference

1   Morley C J, Thornton A J, Cole T J, Hewson P H, Fowler M A 1991 Baby Check: a scoring system to grade the severity of acute systemic illness in babies under 6 months old. Arch Dis Child 66(1):100–105

Further reading

Advanced Life Support Group (eds) 2002 Advanced paediatric life support. The practical approach, 4th edn. BMJ Books, London

Advanced Life Support Group (eds) 2005 Pre-hospital paediatric life support. The practical approach, 2nd edn. Blackwell Publishing, Oxford

American Academy of Pediatrics 2000 Pediatric education for prehospital professionals. Jones and Bartlett, Sudbury, MA.

Department of Health 2003 What to do if you are worried a child is being abused (summary). Crown Publishing, London

Montague A 1996 Legal problems in emergency medicine. Oxford University Press, Oxford

Morley C J, Thornton A J, Cole T J, Hewson P H, Fowler M A. Baby Check. Available online: http://nicutools.org/ (5 Mar 2007)

Fiona Jewkes and Malcolm Woollard

Childhood illness – assessment and management of primary survey negative children

Introduction

This chapter describes the assessment and findings associated with illnesses that commonly affect children. It aims to be a guide to common presentations and treatment rather than a comprehensive review of all paediatric conditions. Chapter 5 describes the identification and initial management of potentially life-threatening problems. Box 6.1 describes the objectives for this chapter.

Secondary survey

A secondary survey will be required for all children who have not required transfer to hospital following the primary survey (see Chapter 5). Its aim is to fully assess the child so that decisions about their future management and disposal can be safely made. The SOAPC system (Box 6.2) can

BOX 6.1 **Chapter objectives**

- To describe the approach to the secondary survey in children and its main features
- To discuss differential diagnosis for children with common presenting symptoms
- To describe the differential diagnosis, management and disposition of children with a range of common conditions
- To review indicators of the need for hospital referral
- To describe the care of common problems affecting technologically assisted children
- To consider the importance of communication in the care of the sick child

BOX 6.2 **SOAPC assessment strategy**

- Subjective assessment
- Objective examination
- Analysis and diagnosis (assessment)
- Plan (treatment and disposal)
- Communication

be used to undertake this survey but is modified to take account of the particular needs of children (see Chapter 5).

Subjective assessment

Most parents and carers will be very sensitive to changes in their children's health. Consequently, if they express concern about their child's wellbeing they are often right. It is important to ask parents or carers what they think the matter is and, if appropriate, what treatment they might be expecting. They may relate treatments that have helped the child during similar illnesses, and this will help to identify the parent's expectations about what they believe is required.

It may be necessary to ask parents what constitutes normal behaviour and appearance for their child, but the patient should always be involved in the discussion. Even toddlers and younger school-age children should be spoken to directly, using language appropriate to their ability to understand. It may be helpful to assess teenagers without parents or guardians present, to encourage them to discuss their illness and any concerns they may have openly.

As well as a detailed history of the presenting complaint, details of past illnesses or operations, medications, and allergies should be sought and recorded, as should the family history. Birth history may also be important, particularly in infants and younger children. On occasion a brief developmental history may also shed light on the problem.

The parents of children with chronic illnesses (such as renal disease) or congenital problems are likely to have considerable expertise about assessment and management of the condition – as indeed may the children themselves. Practitioners should not be dismissive of information provided and suggestions made by 'expert' parents and children. It is important to remember, however, that although they be very knowledgeable about their field of expertise, they are likely to know no more than other people about other medical problems.

Objective examination

Before approaching a child directly, it is a good idea to observe their general behaviour (Fig. 6.1). Are they passive or active? Are they playing normally? Do they pay attention to their surroundings?

When approaching a child, their behaviour should be noted. Is this normal for their age group? Have they reacted to your presence (perhaps by hiding behind the furniture)? Consider the child's general condition – do they appear well cared for, or are they grubby and thin?

The content of the physical examination should be similar to that for an adult, although the order in which each system is assessed may be

Fig. 6.1 A happy, alert baby (reproduced with permission of Dr Claudia Morley).

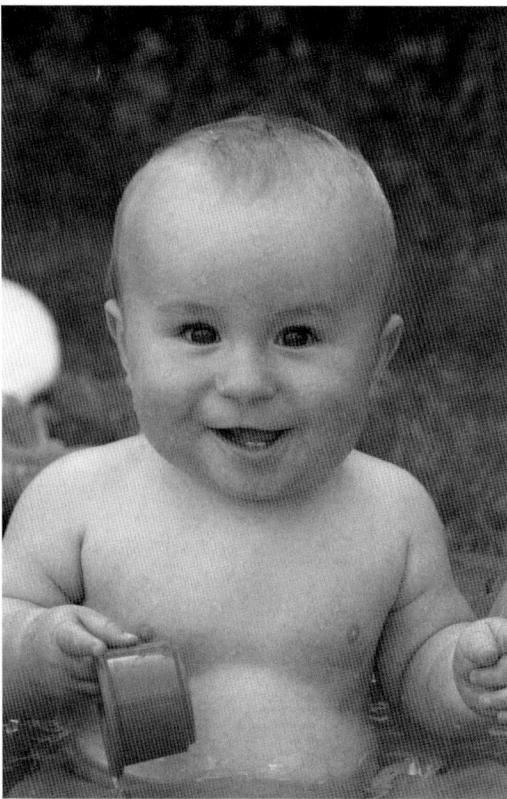

modified depending on the age and behaviour of the child (see Chapter 5). A cardiovascular, respiratory and abdominal examination should be undertaken as appropriate and opportunistically. There are some aspects, however, that are particularly important to the examination of the child.

Skin

The presence of a rash may be significant. The morphology, pattern and distribution should be noted and its significance assessed in the light of the associated symptoms and signs.

Ear, nose and throat

The ears should be examined using an auroscope, and the throat inspected for evidence of tonsillitis or other pathology.

Lymphadenopathy and meningism

Cervical lymphadenopathy is extremely common in upper respiratory tract infections and its presence may lead the child to complain of pain when their neck is flexed. This should not be confused with the neck stiffness seen in meningeal irritation. True meningism may be associated with the child adopting a posture of hyperextension of the head and trunk and the child will be truly unable to flex the neck without stiffness occurring. Meningism may also be associated with a high-pitched cry and patients may present with drowsiness or irritability. Signs of meningism should alert the practitioner to strongly consider meningitis. Lymphadenopathy may also indicate glandular fever, other viral infections, or even relatively rare pathology such as leukaemia. Meningism is often absent in infants with meningitis and in those who have been previously treated with antibiotics (even very small amounts). A lowered threshold for referral is indicated as lumbar puncture may be necessary.

Abdominal examination

Mild splenomegaly is fairly common in viral illnesses but its presence must be noted and the assessment repeated when the child recovers to ensure that it has resolved. The liver may be palpated without difficulty in the young baby but is commonly easily pushed down in conditions where the lungs are hyperinflated such as bronchiolitis. Cardiac failure in children and babies is rare, but must be considered if the baby appears to have an enlarged liver.

Temperature

Taking the child's temperature is of limited value in primary care as the presence or absence of a fever does not confirm or rule out serious disease.

There are various confounding problems, such as whether or not the child has received an antipyretic and what part of the body is used to assess temperature. Indeed authorities still debate what the upper limit of normal is. It is, however, recognised that very young babies (for example, less than 6 months old) who have a significant fever (>38.5 °C) or who are hypothermic (<35 °C) are *more* likely to have serious disease. Young children may sometimes tolerate very high temperatures (>40 °C) with little apparent discomfort or serious pathology. Significant fever can usually be detected, if no thermometer is available, by touching the skin of the child's trunk.

Urine cultures

A sterile urine sample needs to be obtained in any child who is unwell and in whom the cause is not clear. Urinary tract infections are a common cause of febrile convulsions. Urine dip sticks which test for nitrite and leukocytes as well as blood and protein can be helpful as a guide as to whether an infection is present and if positive the urine must be sent for bacteriological diagnosis and antibiotic sensitivity. It is important to obtain urine for culture before starting antibiotics for suspected urinary tract infection. The parent can be instructed to collect the urine before starting antibiotics and store it in the refrigerator until the next day, when the staff at the child's general practice can send it for culture.

It is important not to withhold antibiotics for culture results, particularly in young children. Babies under the age of 6 months in whom there is a high likelihood of urinary tract infection should be referred to hospital the same day, as the risk of renal scarring from infection is high in this age group and intravenous antibiotics are usually employed initially even if the baby seems to be well.

Blood sugar measurement

Whilst blood sugar measurement is essential in all children who have a disturbed conscious level or are diabetic, it need not be done routinely in the child who does not appear to be seriously ill, unless there is a particular reason such as a suspicion of diabetes.

> **TIP**
>
> There are almost no indications for a rectal or vaginal examination in children in the primary care setting

> **TIP**
>
> Children who grab your stethoscope and play with it, and can be made to laugh by wobbling their tummy are not usually seriously ill!

Analysis (differential diagnosis) and treatment and disposal (plan)

Common presentations

The irritable child

A common presentation that can be difficult to address is a baby who is reported to cry excessively. A truly irritable baby dislikes handling and must be assumed to have serious illness and be admitted urgently to hospital. More common is the baby who will not settle or settles only briefly, or the misery of the febrile toddler: these children can cause considerable concern to new parents and healthcare professionals alike but are not necessarily very ill. The cause may be due to a multitude of reasons from significant pathology to poor parenting skills. Even when the practitioner can confidently determine there is no significant clinical problem (difficult at the best of times) admission to hospital or referral for further support should be considered if parents remain anxious.

Abdominal pain

Abdominal pain can also cause diagnostic conundrums. If a child is seriously ill (primary survey positive) he or she should be managed with immediate transfer to hospital and appropriate resuscitative measures. If the child is not seriously ill, the diagnosis can be divided into acute and chronic presentations.

Acute abdominal pain is common. Potential surgical pathology must be excluded and if this is not possible, the child referred for more detailed assessment. Appendicitis may be very difficult to diagnose in small children and must be actively considered. Other serious causes such as intussusception or volvulus may occasionally underlie the acute abdomen. Urinary tract infection must be sought as it often presents non-specifically with abdominal pain with or without urinary symptoms. One of the commoner causes of acute abdominal pain is mesenteric adenitis (acute lymphadenopathy in the abdominal lymph nodes) and a concurrent upper respiratory infection is characteristic. Infective gastroenteritis, Henoch–Schonlein purpura (HSP) and many other disorders all have their own spectrum of associated features and symptoms. If in doubt, refer.

Chronic abdominal pain is also common but more likely to present as a non-urgent complaint, unless the problem is an acute exacerbation of an ongoing problem. Causes are diverse and beyond the scope of this chapter – some of the commoner sources of abdominal pain include urinary tract infection, constipation, abdominal migraine and idiopathic causes (the aptly named 'recurrent abdominal pain of childhood').

The febrile child

Reducing the temperature of febrile children does not have any significant benefit in reducing the length or severity of the associated illness. However simple anti-pyretics, such as paracetamol (known as acetaminophen in the USA) or ibuprofen (which can be used concurrently), can reduce the misery in both child and carer alike (see below).

ENT problems

These are common in children. Infants are obligate nasal breathers up to about 6 months of age. Consequently a blocked nose may result in a significant increase in the work of breathing and may produce difficulty

TIP

Children who have become suddenly and unusually irritable or drowsy and floppy should be considered to be acutely ill until proven otherwise

PITFALL

Infants and toddlers often have a protuberant abdomen – this should not be confused with pathological distension

TIP

Unilateral pain is often a significant finding, and the greater the distance the pain is from the umbilicus the more likely it is to be organic. However, remember that small children localise abdominal pain poorly and will therefore tend to point to the umbilicus as the location wherever the pathology (or even to appear cooperative!)

feeding. Otitis media, presenting with a red and sometimes bulging or perforated eardrum, is a common finding in a child with earache (see Chapter 11). Antibiotics have not been shown to alter the outcome of the disease in the majority of patients, but are still often given. The SIGN guidelines for management of otitis media recommend that antibiotics should not be immediately prescribed, but suggest a 5-day course of amoxicillin should be made available for collection from the GP if the child's condition has not improved after 72 hours. Paracetamol (acetaminophen) and ibuprofen (alone or in combination) usually provide effective symptomatic relief.[1] Otitis externa is less common and usually also presents as earache (which may be severe), with or without a discharge. Antibiotic/steroid ear drops are appropriate.

Foreign bodies may be pushed into the ear by small children or, more commonly, into the nose, and should be sought in the presence of a snuffly child without symptoms of illness. The throat should be carefully examined in all sick children unless epiglottitis or croup is suspected. Streptococcal infections and glandular fever can cause petechial rashes on the palate, ulcers may indicate a Coxsackie virus infection, and Koplik's spots are indicative of measles (which is rare nowadays). Swollen red tonsils, with or without exudates, and accompanied by flulike symptoms suggest tonsillitis or possibly glandular fever. Unilateral enlargement may suggest a peri-tonsillar abscess.

Respiratory problems

Respiratory problems account for approximately 40% of children admitted to hospital, with the majority being for asthma (see Chapter 4). Croup is usually viral and presents with a seal-like bark with or without systemic illness or associated stridor. There may be other symptoms of upper respiratory tract infection including fever but the child is not generally very unwell. Sudden onset, short history, drooling due to pain and a very toxic child support the diagnosis of the now rare epiglottitis, which should be considered to be immediately life threatening.

Wheezing in babies may be due to a variety of causes, two of the commoner ones being asthma or bronchiolitis, the latter resulting in the hospitalisation of 2–3% of infants each year. Bronchiolitis is seasonal, occurring in the winter months and classically fine inspiratory crepitations may be heard on auscultation. Sudden or recurrent apnoea may occur in small babies with bronchiolitis, and infants with compromised immune systems, congenital heart disease or chronic lung disease. In older children asthma is the most likely cause of wheezing. Anaphylaxis should be considered as an unlikely possibility in a child with a first presentation of wheezing, as should the possibility of inhalation of a foreign body.

Significant respiratory tract infections, such as pneumonia, also occur in children and can result in hypoxia, respiratory failure, septicaemia, hypoglycaemia, or dehydration due to the inability to feed.

Illnesses rarely requiring hospital admission

Table 6.1 describes common illnesses and presentations in children that rarely require hospital admission. Upper respiratory tract infections are particularly common in children, but foreign bodies in the airway should always be considered as a possible explanation of mild stridor or wheeze in otherwise well children. Children are also susceptible to a wide range of viral infections, many of which present with rashes of various descriptions.

Symptomatic treatment for pain or fever consists of paracetamol or ibuprofen. Both drugs can be used together for their synergistic effect, 'staggering' the doses if required. Encourage maintenance of an intake of (preferably) clear fluids.

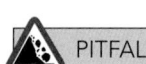 **PITFALL**

Ibuprofen is contraindicated in children with asthma

The choice of antibiotic and some other treatments may vary according to local protocols or where complications occur. Antibiotics should **not** be given blindly in a child who is generally unwell or has a fever of unknown cause. This may make the subsequent diagnosis of serious disease such as meningitis very difficult and thus be a risky strategy overall.

To hospitalise or not?

In many situations it can be difficult to decide whether to send children to hospital because they fall neither into the category of 'primary survey positive patients' nor that of the relatively well child described in Table 6.1. The signs of serious illness in children are subtle and it is usually wise to err on the side of safety and ask for a second opinion if in doubt. However, some evidence-based pointers that may be helpful in deciding whether hospital referral is necessary are given below.[2]

General

- Babies less than 2 months old
- Co-morbidity with a chronic disorder, e.g. congenital heart disease
- Lack of social support – parents unable to cope, previous child abuse

Upper airway obstruction

- Signs of severe respiratory distress
- Signs of serious illness
- Strong suspicion of aspiration
- Stertorous (snoring) breathing

Wheezing and coughing

- Suspicion of foreign body
- Child under 2 months old
- Significant respiratory distress
- History of apnoeic attack

Common conditions	Subjective findings	Objective findings*	Plan	Disposition
TABLE 6.1 Diagnosis, treatment and disposition of common childhood illnesses not requiring hospital admission				
General				
Fever	Hot and unwell Miserable May be off food/ fluids	Depends on cause (must be sought and found)	Exclude serious cause Symptomatic treatment Cause must be sought (including urine culture if no other cause found) Do not give antibiotics if cause unknown	Care at home, refer for further investigations if cause cannot be identified and child significantly unwell or serious cause cannot be excluded
Vomiting	Frequency ?blood ?tolerating clear fluids

? bile stained | Rule out: – dehydration – other sign of infection – surgical pathology | Exclude abdominal or other serious pathology If tolerating clear fluids, encourage clear fluids till improving then solid diet Do not give anti-emetics | Care at home unless very unwell/ dehydrated or significant pathology cannot be excluded |
| Diarrhoea | Need description ?blood, ?slime, ?watery, ?amount, ?colour May be vomiting or anorexic | Rule out: – abdominal abnormalities – signs of dehydration – other signs of infection Mild fever may be present | Encourage clear/ electrolyte replacement fluids to re-hydrate only Exclude occult infection and dehydration Exclude other abdominal pathology Continue breastfeeding throughout Recommence solids and formula feeds after re-hydrating Avoid foods high in fat or simple sugars Do not give anti-diarrhoeal agents | Care at home unless very unwell/ dehydrated or history of bloody diarrhoea, or significant pathology cannot be excluded |

(*Continued*)

TABLE 6.1 Diagnosis, treatment and disposition of common childhood illnesses not requiring hospital admission—Cont'd

Common conditions	Subjective findings	Objective findings*	Plan	Disposition
Respiratory				
Upper respiratory tract infection	Cough 'Cold' Sore throat Snuffly Hot and miserable May be off food/fluids	Inflamed throat Otitis media Coryza Chest clear Fever	Symptomatic treatment No antibiotics Review if fluid intake poor	Care at home Antipyretics
Croup (mild)	Barking cough Noisy breathing May be worse at night	Barking cough May have mild stridor Child not distressed May have other URT signs Do not examine throat Mild fever possible	Nebulised budesonide or oral dexamethasone Do not examine throat	Care at home unless systemically unwell or deteriorating
Asthma (mild)	Wheeze Cough May be URTI	Bilateral wheeze Good air entry May be mildly tachypnoeic Child not distressed	Adjustment of dose of bronchodilator Check technique of administration using spacer Oral (soluble if necessary) prednisolone	Care at home unless no response to treatment, deteriorating. Lowered threshold for admission if history of previous ITU admission
Bronchiolitis (mild)	URT symptoms followed by lower respiratory symptoms	Not distressed Mild tachypnoea Mild fever possible Bilateral inspiratory fine crackles and wheeze	Symptomatic treatment	Care at home; consider need for follow-up visit and encourage recall if condition deteriorates (especially reluctance to feed or breathing difficulty). Very low threshold for admission in babies under 2 months old

TABLE 6.1 Diagnosis, treatment and disposition of common childhood illnesses not requiring hospital admission—Cont'd

Common conditions	Subjective findings	Objective findings*	Plan	Disposition
ENT/eyes				
Conjunctivitis	Sore gritty eyes Normal visual acuity	Mildly inflamed conjunctiva, often bilaterally Sometimes purulent discharge	Regular cleaning with cooled boiled water Antibiotic eye drops	Care at home unless very severe in neonate
Foreign body	History of witnessed insertion of object in nose, ear 'Missing' object Sudden respiratory distress	Foreign body visible Stridor Wheeze Unequal air entry	May be possible to remove – if not refer to appropriate specialist	Care at home if object removed, otherwise refer to A&E Do not attempt to remove blindly if lodged in pharynx
Tonsillitis	Sore throat Systemically unwell Sore neck Difficulty swallowing	Swollen inflamed tonsils Exudate Lymphadenopathy Fever	Mild – symptomatic treatment, otherwise penicillin (unless allergic when use suitable alternative) for 10 days and symptomatic treatment	Care at home with advice to recall if swallowing becomes impossible or airway becomes noisy
Teething	Miserable	Teeth erupting	Symptomatic treatment	Care at home
Otitis media	Miserable	Inflamed ear drum ± perforation Fever possible	Symptomatic treatment Consider antibiotics if very severe or if eardrum is perforated	Care at home If eardrum perforated, refer to GP for review and keep ear dry

(*Continued*)

TABLE 6.1 Diagnosis, treatment and disposition of common childhood illnesses not requiring hospital admission—Cont'd

Common conditions	Subjective findings	Objective findings*	Plan	Disposition
Skin and viral rashes				
Chicken pox (uncomplicated)	Mild URTI symptoms Rash	Blistering rash in crops, most marked on trunk Mild fever	Symptomatic treatment	Care at home
Scabies	Itchy rash	Itchy papules, may be more generalised than in adults, with some 'tracks'	Non-urgent referral to GP	Care at home and non-urgent referral to GP
Impetigo	Crusting rash	Yellow/golden crusting spreading rash May occasionally be systemically unwell May be painful, especially if secondary infection	Systemic antibiotics unless very tiny lesion when topical antibiotics may be tried	Care at home Advise on reducing spread to other family members
Mumps (un-complicated)	Swollen neck Difficulty opening mouth and swallowing Mild fever/malaise	Parotid swelling Loss of palpable angle of mandible	Symptomatic treatment	Care at home
Rubella	Fine pink rash May be very slightly unwell	Fine macular rash Posterior cervical lymphadenopathy Minimal systemic upset	Symptomatic treatment Check no contact with pregnant adult is likely	Care at home

TABLE 6.1 Diagnosis, treatment and disposition of common childhood illnesses not requiring hospital admission—Cont'd

Common conditions	Subjective findings	Objective findings*	Plan	Disposition
Roseola infantum	High fever >38.5 °C) which settles when rash comes out	Discrete rash which may coalesce May be oedema of eyelids Fever	Symptomatic treatment	Care at home
Measles (un-complicated)	Upper respiratory symptoms Rash	Unwell child Koplik's spots early in illness Typical rash Upper respiratory tract signs No sign of complications (e.g. pneumonia)	Symptomatic treatment	Care at home Notifiable disease
Neurology				
Increase in seizures	In child known to have seizures	Infection or any obvious cause Recent change in medication dose; not taking medication or malabsorbing (e.g. GI upset)	Look for infection	Refer to GP if not currently seizing and otherwise well; refer to A&E if currently seizing or seizures very frequent (see chapter on primary survey positive children)
Head injury (mild)	No symptoms	May be bruising	Rule out significant mechanism of injury If no loss of consciousness, persistent vomiting (≥2 vomits), unusual drowsiness, or visual disturbance since injury, advise that treatment should be sought if these symptoms present	Care at home in the absence of history of loss of consciousness and significant symptoms; advise recall if symptoms present Provide written head injury instructions

(*Continued*)

TABLE 6.1 Diagnosis, treatment and disposition of common childhood illnesses not requiring hospital admission—Cont'd

Common conditions	Subjective findings	Objective findings*	Plan	Disposition
Headache	Ask for type, when it occurs in day, associated features	Exclude serious infection Past history & investigations	Look for signs of raised intra-cranial pressure and meningitis	If child well with no signs of meningitis, provide symptomatic treatment and refer to GP Arrange urgent review if unwell or condition worsens
Febrile convulsions	Fever, child known to have febrile convulsions	Fever Infection Usual age range approx. 6 months to 6 years	Locate source of infection and treat, referring to hospital if serious cause found or if no cause found Check blood sugar	Care at home for simple febrile convulsions, provided – this is not the first fit – it is a simple convulsion – the cause of the fever has been identified and is benign – no more than one fit in a 24-hour period – the parents are confident about caring for the child – advise on treatment/antipyretics
Abdomen Abdominal pain (colicky)	May be irritable	Rule out surgical problem abnormalities Look for associated features (see above)	Exclude appendicitis, obstruction or other pathology Symptomatic treatment	If child is completely well, refer to GP. If child is unwell or parents are concerned, refer urgently to GP or hospital

TABLE 6.1 Diagnosis, treatment and disposition of common childhood illnesses not requiring hospital admission—Cont'd

Common conditions	Subjective findings	Objective findings*	Plan	Disposition
Dysuria	Complaining of pain when passing urine	Balanitis possible Rule out renal tenderness Check otherwise well or minimum systemic upset	Mild balanitis can be treated with salt baths If balanitis is severe will require antibiotics If no balanitis check urine culture and treat for urinary tract infection till results of culture available	Care at home; refer for further investigations if no cause found

*Only some may be present and only most common are listed

Febrile seizures

- First febrile convulsion
- Infants less than 18 months old with fever or history of prior treatment with antibiotics
- Complex or focal seizure
- Drowsiness before seizure
- Contact with GP/A&E in previous 24 hours
- Tense fontanelle or possible neck stiffness
- No focus of infection
- Parental anxiety

Afebrile seizures

- Depressed conscious level more than 1 hour after fit
- New neurological signs
- Age less than 1 year (unless seizures are part of the child's chronic condition)
- Signs of raised intracranial pressure
- Signs of meningism
- Unwell with no obvious cause
- Signs of aspiration
- Parental anxiety

TIP

If in doubt, ask for help!

Diarrhoea and vomiting

- Doubt in diagnosis (possible underlying pathology)

Poor fluid intake or vomiting, particularly if in association with:

- Age less than 6 months
- More than 4 vomits per day
- More than 8 liquid stools per day
- No diagnosis

PITFALL

Children aged less than 1 year or those who have received any prior antibiotics may not have neck stiffness in the presence of meningitis

PITFALL

The absence of a non-blanching rash does not rule out meningococcal septicaemia

TIP

Always be sure you are satisfied that any ill child does not have meningitis, appendicitis or urinary tract infection as all three are common and relatively easily missed. If you are not certain, refer

Findings for exclusion if hospital attendance is not considered appropriate

Viral infections that commonly result in childhood illnesses may occasionally be associated with serious complications. Mumps, measles, chicken pox and rubella can all result in inflammation and damage of a number of organs. Complications can include meningitis, encephalitis, hepatitis and pancreatitis. Children presenting with these conditions will require urgent referral for supportive treatment.

Always consider meningitis in children with flu-like illness who have deteriorated rapidly over 4–6 hours.

Children with evidence of dehydration and/or reduced urine output, regardless of cause, may require intravenous fluids including dextrose. Abdominal pain will require referral if significant pathology cannot be ruled out.

Disposition flow chart

Figure 6.2 shows the decision-making process for determining the urgency of care required and the appropriate disposition for children with a range of presenting problems.

Technologically assisted children

Children requiring technological support such as assisted ventilation and tube feeding are increasingly being cared for at home. Pre-hospital practitioners called to assist such children may be unfamiliar with this equipment but should be aware of the small number of interventions that can be appropriately made in the out-of-hospital setting. Remember that parents, carers and even the child may be able to offer expert advice themselves, and should also be able to provide contact details for professional advice.

Tracheostomy tubes

In the event that a tracheostomy tube becomes obstructed, the following approach should be adopted:

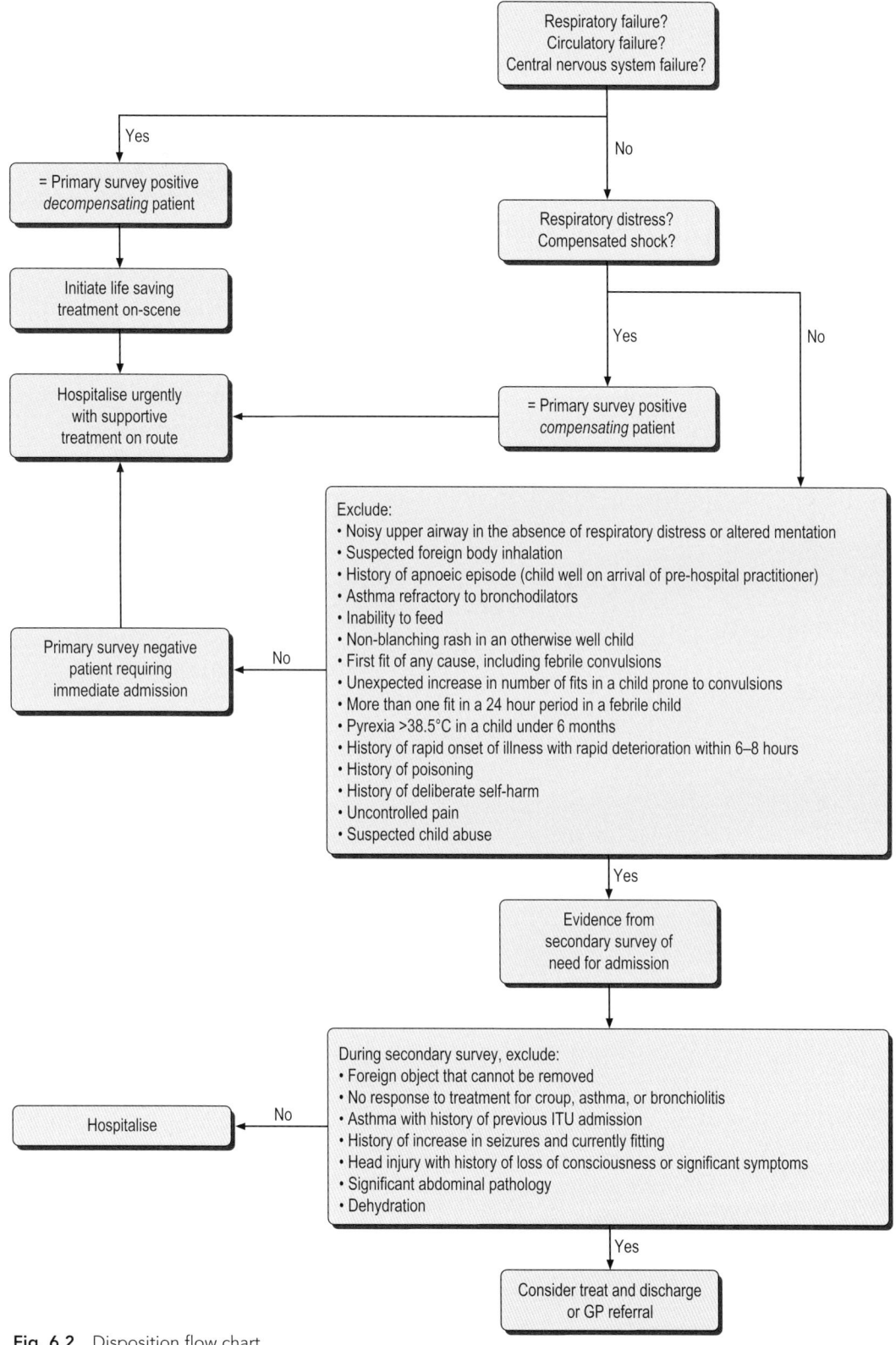

Fig. 6.2 Disposition flow chart.

1. Confirm the tube is correctly positioned
2. Remove the speech-cap from fenestrated tubes
3. Suction the tube to remove secretions (use the tube's obturator to clear it if suction is not available)
4. If a fenestrated tube is being used, replace the tube liner with a new one
5. Remove the entire tracheostomy tube and replace
6. Ventilate to confirm correct position and patency.

Ventilated children

In the event of failure of a ventilator, confirm the problem is not due to airway obstruction. In the event of genuine failure of the device, assist breathing with a self-inflating bag with supplementary oxygen and transport to hospital. If an adjustable automatic ventilator is available on the ambulance, set this to deliver a tidal volume of 7–10 ml/kg to replace the work of the child's normal ventilator and limit maximum airway pressure to 20 cmH$_2$O initially, increasing carefully until the chest moves.

Central venous catheters

Central venous catheters may be used for feeding, dialysis or administration of medication. If a catheter becomes dislodged, the wound should be dressed, and direct pressure applied as necessary to control bleeding. If bleeding occurs through a break in the catheter, the tube should be clamped proximally. The child's hospital team should be contacted to arrange a review.

Infection at the insertion site will present as local reddening, tenderness, or a purulent discharge, which may also be associated with systemic signs of infection. Infection of the catheter itself will often present with signs of a non-specific serious infection and septicaemia. The catheter should not be used and the child referred to their medical team. Seriously damaged catheters are likely to require replacement whereas every effort is usually made to preserve the catheter in infection, if possible. Children with signs of septicaemia will require urgent antibiotic and supportive therapy.

In the event that a tube is obstructed, the child should be referred to hospital. The tube may be subsequently thrombolysed or, as a last resort, replaced. Fluid should not be forced down the tube. Hypoglycaemia and dehydration should be considered and managed in children dependent on the tube for nutrition.

Air embolism may occur as a result of incorrect flushing procedures or a mishap (usually during haemodialysis), and will present as coughing, dyspnoea and chest pain. The tube must be clamped and the child transferred urgently to hospital in a head-down, left-lateral position, with high concentration oxygen therapy. CPR may be necessary. The A&E department must be alerted.

Ventriculoperitoneal shunts

Ventriculoperitoneal (VP) shunts are surgically implanted in children with hydrocephalus to allow drainage of cerebrospinal fluid. Obstruction of the shunt will result in raised intra-cranial pressure, the signs of which will include altered affect, high pitched cry, fitting, and falling level of consciousness, similar to the presentation of meningitis. Children with evidence of an obstructed shunt require urgent hospital admission. The presence of Cushing's triad (bradycardia, hypertension and Cheyne–Stokes ventilation) indicates the ICP is so high that brainstem impairment is occurring and is a critical situation. Supportive care should be provided during transfer to the hospital. If the child is very ill this will include airway care and high concentration oxygen therapy. Controlled hyperventilation (at a rate of 5 inflations per minute above the child's normal respiratory rate) should be used only in children with signs of Cushing's triad. Most children present sooner than this because parents have been trained to look for warning signs (and sometimes to check the shunt) and less rapid transfer will be more suitable.

Infection around the shunt may also occur, resulting in altered affect, headache, fever, and refusal to take feeds. Septicaemia can also result from shunt infections resulting in a lowered level of consciousness and shock. Urgent transfer to hospital with supportive and antibiotic therapy is indicated.

Feeding tubes

Feeding tubes may be positioned through the nose or rarely, the mouth, or be implanted through the abdominal wall. Most parents or carers (and indeed some children themselves!) in the UK are trained to replace nasogastric tubes, or local arrangements will have been made for a healthcare professional (for example at the community hospital or a community nurse) to do this. Hospital admission is therefore not usually necessary. Percutaneous tubes will usually require reinsertion in hospital as a matter of some urgency and the relevant unit should be contacted to arrange this.

Infected catheter sites should be cleaned and the hospital contacted to discuss review and to decide on appropriate antibiotic treatment. It is not necessary to discontinue use.

If correct placement of an enteral feeding tube cannot be confirmed, discontinue any infusion until the situation can be resolved by testing with litmus paper, which will show the presence of acid if the tube is in the stomach.

Table 6.2 provides a quick reference guide to managing a number of common problems.

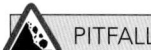

PITFALL

If a child is on continuous enteral or intravenous feeds, remember to monitor for hypoglycaemia if it is necessary to discontinue an infusion

TABLE 6.2 Management of common problems in technologically assisted children

Device	Problem(s)	Solution(s)
Tracheostomy tube	Obstruction	1. Confirm tube is correctly positioned 2. Remove the speech-cap from fenestrated tubes 3. Suction the tube to remove secretions (use the tube's obturator if suction is not available) 4. If a fenestrated tube is being used, replace the tube liner with a new one 5. Remove the tracheostomy tube and replace 6. Ventilate to confirm correct position and patency
Home ventilator	Failure	1. Confirm the problem is not due to airway obstruction 2. Assist breathing with a self-inflating bag with supplementary oxygen and transport to hospital
Central venous catheter	Catheter dislodged	1. Dress the wound 2. Apply direct pressure to control bleeding 3. Contact the hospital and inform the child's medical team
	Broken/perforated catheter	1. Clamp catheter tube proximal to break to prevent air embolus 2. Transfer to hospital
	Infection at insertion site or possible infected catheter	1. Discontinue use 2. If the child is very ill, transfer treating A, B, C as per primary survey positive patients. Do not remove the catheter! 3. Mild local infection will also need hospital review
	Obstruction	Contact hospital and arrange review and discuss need for rehydration/prevention of hypoglycaemia (will depend on the purpose of the tube)
	Air embolism (following incorrect flushing technique)	1. Clamp the tube 2. Transfer urgently to hospital in a head-down, left-lateral position 3. Give high concentration oxygen 4. Provide CPR if necessary
Ventriculoperitoneal (VP) shunts	Obstruction (causing raised intracranial pressure)	1. If child seriously ill treat ABCs and transfer immediately to hospital 2. Use controlled hyperventilation (at a rate of 5 inflations per minute above the child's normal respiratory rate) if Cushing's triad present; otherwise transfer urgently
	Infection/septicaemia	1. Transfer urgently to hospital; manage as meningitis 2. Consider need for supportive therapy

TABLE 6.2 Management of common problems in technologically assisted children—Cont'd		
Device	Problem(s)	Solution(s)
Nasogastric or percutaneous feeding tubes (PEGs)	Dislodged	1. Discontinue use 2. Remove nasogastric tube if not already out 3. Either replace or arrange transfer to healthcare personnel who usually replace tube (many parents and some children will replace nasogastric tubes themselves) 4. If a PEG is dislodged, arrange transfer to hospital for review by the child's medical team
	Infected site	Clean and dress the site; arrange hospital review

Communication and follow-up

Parents do not ask for help unless they are worried. Provide a simple explanation of your findings and of the implications of these for their child's health. Offer reassurance and clear parameters for re-contacting the service if things are not going according to plan. Where appropriate provide written advice. Always seek help from someone more expert or the hospital if unsure.

Acknowledgements

Suggestions made by Peter Driscoll and Jim Wardrope resulted in improvements to an earlier draft of this chapter. Our thanks to them and to Fiona Mair, who generously provided her time and expertise to source the pictures.

References

1 Scottish Intercollegiate Guidelines Network 2003 Diagnosis and management of childhood otitis media in primary care. Section 3: Medical treatment. SIGN, Edinburgh. Available online: http://www.sign.ac.uk/guidelines/fulltext/66/section3.html (5 Mar 2007)
2 Paediatric Accident and Emergency Research Group 2002 Evidence based guidelines for acute management with breathing difficulty, diarrhoea & vomiting, post-seizure. Children Nationwide, Cheltenham

Further reading

Advanced Life Support Group (eds) 2002 Advanced paediatric life support. The practical approach, 4th edn. BMJ Books, London

Advanced Life Support Group (eds) 2005 Pre-hospital paediatric life support. The practical approach, 2nd edn. Blackwell Publishing, Oxford

American Academy of Pediatrics 2000 Pediatric education for prehospital professionals. Jones and Bartlett, Sudbury, MA

Behrman R E, Kliegman R, Nelson T 1990 Essentials of paediatrics. WB Saunders, Philadelphia, PA

Gill D, O'Brien N 2003 Paediatric clinical examination made easy, 4th edn. Churchill Livingstone, Edinburgh

Morley C J, Thornton A J, Cole T J, Hewson P H, Fowler M A 2000 Baby Check. Available online: http://nicutools.org (5 Mar 2007)

Ninnis N, Glennie L 2004 Lessons from research for doctors in training. Meningitis Research Foundation, Bristol

Appendix: pharmacopoeia

Table 6.3 describes the indications, contraindications and doses of drugs commonly used to treat illness in childhood.

TABLE 6.3 Drugs commonly used in childhood illnesses

Drug name	Indications	Contraindications	Dose
Epinephrine (adrenaline)	Anaphylaxis associated with wheeze or respiratory distress (including cyanosis) unrelieved by salbutamol OR stridor OR clinical signs of shock (systolic BP <90 mmHg)	None	6–11 years: 250 µg (0.25 ml of 1:1000) IM 6 months–5 years: 120 µg (0.12 ml of 1:1000) IM <6 months: 50 µg (0.05 ml of 1:1000) IM All ages: repeat after 5 minutes if necessary
Epinephrine (adrenaline)	Croup associated with severe respiratory distress	None	1 ml 1:1000 via nebuliser once only whilst definitive care arranged

TABLE 6.3 Drugs commonly used in childhood illnesses—Cont'd

Drug name	Indications	Contraindications	Dose
Benzylpenicillin	Meningococcal septicaemia (also see cefotaxime)	Confirmed penicillin allergy	For IV/IO use, dilute 600 mg in 10 ml; for IM, dilute 600 mg in 2 ml Less than one year 300 mg (5 ml IV/IO or 1 ml IM) 1–9 years 600 mg (10 ml IV/IO or 2 ml IM) > 9 years and adult 1.2 g (20 ml IV/IO or 4 ml IM)
Budesonide	Croup	Less than 3 months old	2 mg via nebuliser, once only
Cefotaxime	Meningococcal septicaemia	Allergy	80 mg/kg IV/IO
Dexamethasone syrup	Croup	None	0.15 mg/kg PO
Dextrose 10%	Hypoglycaemia	None	5 ml/kg IV/IO, titrated to blood sugar
Diazepam	Continuous or recurrent fits	None	Rectal: 0–1 years 2.5 mg; 1–3 years 5 mg; 4–12 years 10 mg IV: 250–400 µg/kg All ages: repeat if required after 5 mins
Hydrocortisone	Anaphylaxis; asthma	None	4 mg/kg IV
Ibuprofen	Fever and mild to moderate pain	Known sensitivity Asthma	10 mg/kg up to tds PO
Ipratropium bromide	Asthma/bronchiolitis	None	Up to 7 years, 125 µg > 7 years 250 µg via nebuliser
Morphine	Moderate to severe pain	Known sensitivity to opiates Respiratory depression, hypotension, or reduced GCS (<12)	IV: 0.1 mg/kg, repeated at 5-min intervals to a maximum dose of 0.2 mg/kg. Use half dose in children <1 year old
Naloxone	Reversal of opiate overdose	None	10 µg/kg IV/IM followed by 100 µg/kg titrated to effect

(Continued)

TABLE 6.3 Drugs commonly used in childhood illnesses—Cont'd			
Drug name	Indications	Contraindications	Dose
Paracetamol suspension or soluble tablets	Fever and mild to moderate pain	Under 2 months	15 mg/kg (maximum single dose 1 g) PO 4–6-hourly
Prednisolone soluble tablets	Exacerbations of asthma	None	1 mg/kg (maximum single dose 60 mg) PO, bd for 5 days
Salbutamol	Asthma/bronchiolitis	None	<1 year 2.5 mg nebulised (if ineffective do not repeat) 1–5 years 2.5 mg repeated at 15 min intervals, titrated to effect >5 years 5 mg repeated at 15 min intervals, titrated to effect
Fucidic acid eye drops	Eye infection – for prophylaxis or treatment	Allergy	Twice daily in the affected eye

Note: known allergy to any of the drugs or constituents is a contraindication in all cases

John Hall and Peter Driscoll

Nausea, vomiting and fever

Introduction

Nausea, vomiting and fever are extremely common presenting complaints in community emergency medicine. They are often symptoms of a minor, self-limiting illness but can also be an early, or only, marker of an underlying, potentially life-threatening medical condition. Box 7.1 shows the objectives of this chapter.

BOX 7.1 Chapter objectives

- Perform a primary survey to identify and treat any life-threatening problem
- Identify key factors in the history and examination (as part of the secondary survey) which will be needed to identify the severity of the underlying condition as well as its possible cause
- To consider a list of differential diagnoses
- To introduce the concept of 'little sick/big sick'
- Discuss treatment based on likely diagnoses and whether home or hospital management is appropriate
- Consider the need and practicality of follow-up if not admitted

Primary survey

On first contact with the patient an assessment needs to be made as to whether they are primary survey positive. If so the person requires immediate appropriate treatment and rapid transfer to hospital (see Chapter 2).

The primary survey box from Chapter 3 (Chest pain) is repeated here as a refresher and is also slightly expanded to include further important triggers for these symptoms (Box 7.2).

Since the signs/symptoms discussed in this chapter span the entire age spectrum some of the parameters will need to be age adjusted. Those parameters in Box 7.2 requiring adjustment are asterisked. Table 7.1 sets out an evidence based paediatric adjusted physiological range for these parameters in children who are OK even though they may be distressed or unhappy.[1] As such they differ from the values derived from children who are behaving normally. Child blood pressure is notoriously difficult to take and requires special equipment rarely carried outside hospital.

BOX 7.2 Primary survey (adult)

If any observations below are present then treat immediately and transfer to hospital:
- Airway obstruction
- Respiratory rate <10 or >29*
- O_2 sats <93%
- Pulse <50 or >120*
- Systolic BP < 90 mmHg
- Glasgow coma score (GCS) <12
- Unexplained neurological signs
- Unexplained rash

TABLE 7.1 Paediatric physiological values		
Age (years)	Pulse rate	Respiratory rate
<2	90–180	20–50
2–5	80–160	15–40
6–12	70–140	10–30

It is unlikely to be abnormal unless other, easier to assess, parameters are affected.

If the patient is primary survey positive they will require immediate treatment appropriate to their findings (see Chapter 2). According to local guidelines this may include administering IM/IV/IO antibiotics and fluids if bacterial meningitis or meningococcal septicaemia is suspected.

If immediate transfer to hospital is indicated then the airway should be secured if necessary, respiration assisted as appropriate and IV access/fluids gained in transit unless the journey time/distance or the patient's condition mandates otherwise.

In many ways finding something requiring urgent transfer to hospital makes management relatively easy – it is often not even necessary to make an accurate diagnosis of the underlying condition. In practice, however, the majority of patients seen with the symptoms dealt with in this chapter will not fall into this category and a more detailed assessment will be needed.[2]

> **TIP**
>
> Before proceeding further with the discussion of the primary survey negative patient's take the opportunity to re-read Chapters 2 and 6

Secondary survey

The vast majority of patients who show no primary survey positive signs will have relatively minor, self-limiting illnesses. A small minority, however, can rapidly deteriorate and may die. It is therefore essential to take a precise history and perform an adequate examination of all patients with these symptoms/signs.

The concept of 'little sick/big sick' is very useful in deciding whether a patient is sufficiently ill to require active intervention or not. Unfortunately it is mainly a concept based on the practitioner's experience but there are certain features that are helpful.

■ *Little sick – unwell*
  ■ look and sound alright
  ■ behave normally for age/time of day

- ABC and level of consciousness (LOC) within normal range for age
- no obvious warning signs
- been going on for a while
- possibly some improvement
- *Big sick – ill*
  - look and sound ill
  - behave abnormally for age/time of day
  - ABC/LOC may be outside normal range
  - warning signs may be present
  - 'gut instinct'

The above lists seem obvious but things are often not as simple as they appear.

Nausea and vomiting

Nausea is a non-specific term usually referring to feeling unwell for any reason. Its generality makes it an unhelpful diagnostic symptom. Vomiting is more precise and may or may not be associated with nausea. Table 7.2 lists the subjective and objective information that needs to be elicited from the patient presenting with nausea or vomiting.

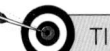

TIP

Elderly patients with seemingly minor cellulitis can have significant systemic symptoms

PITFALL

Even viral illnesses can kill!

Analysis

Nausea and vomiting with no other significant features are usually due to a minor viral illness. Unfortunately they may also be associated with the early stages of a multiplicity of illnesses including brain tumours, balance mechanism dysfunction, poisoning by food or drugs (especially overuse of alcohol!), intra-abdominal pathology and serious life-threatening infections.

However, if no adverse features have been found during the examination and the patient is alert, apyrexial and showing no sign of rapid progression of symptoms then no further specific treatment needs to be given.

Any abnormalities discovered may be treated, referred or transferred to hospital depending upon local protocols and resource availability. Box 7.3 lists common and less common causes of nausea and vomiting.

RED FLAG

Any patient showing evidence of altered level of consciousness, dehydration, neurological symptoms/signs, unusual or uncertain rash, significant abdominal pain/distension or signs of jaundice should be transferred to hospital for further investigation[3]

TABLE 7.2 Information that needs to be elicited from the patient presenting with nausea or vomiting

Subjective	Objective
The symptom How long has the symptom been present? How long have the symptoms been a problem? How often has the person vomited in the past few hours? Is there any blood or mucus in the vomit? What colour is the vomit? **Associated symptoms** Is there any associated pain? Where is it and does it radiate anywhere? Is there any diarrhoea? If so is there any blood or mucus in it? **Possible infective contacts/travel** Does anyone else in the family have the same problems? What does the patient/family think is the cause? Have they been abroad, if so where? **Past history** Is there a significant past medical history of similar episodes or recent illness/surgery? Is the patient immunocompromised by pre-existing illness or recent treatment? They will usually have a letter from hospital explaining the risks, if this is likely Has the patient taken any drugs prescribed or otherwise? If not should they have? Is the patient pregnant? If so how pregnant?	**General** Baseline vital signs are measured Is there any evidence of dehydration? Look in the mouth/ears. Check lymph glands Look for evidence of jaundice Is there rash or widespread muscle tenderness? **Systems exam as indicated by history** *Neurological* Is there any headache, visual symptoms, altered level of consciousness, or neurological signs including abnormal tone in children? *Chest* As indicated by the history *Abdomen* Is there any abdominal pain? If so the abdomen should be palpated and listened to for signs of bowel disease or obstruction and the renal angles palpated for tenderness Are there any urinary or gynaecological symptoms, e.g. dysuria and frequency or vaginal discharge? **Tests** Check a urine specimen if possible (Nephur test or Combistix) checking for nitrites or cells Check a BM test in the very young and the elderly even if there is no history of diabetes

---

BOX 7.3 Causes of nausea and vomiting

Common
- Gastroenteritis
- Viral illness
- Pregnancy
- Associated with acute abdomen

Not uncommon
- Bacterial infections, pneumonia, pyelonephritis
- Renal and biliary colic
- Hyperglycaemia
- Intestinal obstruction
- Migraine

Uncommon
- Septicaemia
- Raised intracranial pressure
- Renal failure
- Acute glaucoma

Plan

If the likely diagnosis is a non-specific viral illness and the patient can be left at home (assuming there is someone to care for them or they are capable of looking after themselves) then symptomatic treatment should be offered.

It used to be held that, assuming no evidence of dehydration is present, at any age a period of 24 hours without food would reduce the overall duration of the symptoms. Recent work[4] would now indicate that at least in children a sensible diet can be continued at all times as long as hydration continues to be maintained. Fluids should continue in small regular amounts at all times – flat, normal cola or lemonade is usually a very palatable option for patients over one year old. Adults over 16 years may be given an anti-emetic (IM or buccal) according to protocol. However if this is given within 12 hours of the onset of symptoms it can extend the duration of symptoms by altering the body's natural reaction to the gastrointestinal irritant.

Communication

An explanation of the likelihood, possibilities and options with the patient and carers has an important therapeutic effect. Allaying unnecessary anxieties can be very useful in allowing the patient to manage the illness.

If the patient is to be left alone then he/she or the carer should be given advice on what to do and who to contact if things do not improve and especially if they worsen. Alternatively a review by phone or in person should be arranged.

Fever

This will be present to some extent in almost every episode of ill health from whatever cause, either as a primary or secondary event. It is therefore of limited value in assessing the nature of the illness and is only slightly more helpful in gauging its severity.

Generally speaking it is true that increased temperature (>38°C) is related to some degree of infection and statistically will normally be viral. However the temperature may be a response to the primary infection, as in flu-like illnesses, or may be a response to secondary infection from the primary cause, as in peritonitis from a ruptured appendix. It must also be remembered that non-infective inflammatory or allergic conditions of many types (inflammatory bowel disease, hay fever, lymphomas) will often present with a fever – sometimes as the only initial symptom. It is also important to remember that the high temperature itself may be the illness. Heat exhaustion or heat stroke can be very serious indeed and require specific treatment, though usually the circumstances of the consultation will lead one to the diagnosis.

If the presence of a fever is not particularly helpful as a diagnostic tool then is there anything about it that can be helpful? There is evidence that a rapidly rising temperature or a temperature >39°C are more likely to be associated with significant bacterial causes requiring further investigation and possible admission.[5,6] Much of this evidence comes from research in A&E departments. This is a pre-selected group of patients and while the findings may not be fully applicable to the pre-hospital setting it is still a useful guide. From a practical perspective it is difficult to judge the rate of temperature rise pre-hospital. It requires you to spend 30 minutes or more with the patient or return and review fairly soon.

Higher temperatures in the very young or very old are more often associated with significant underlying illness and are more likely to require hospital admission and investigation.[3,5,6] In addition these age groups tend to have associated carers who can provide useful information regarding the underlying cause and their ability to cope with the illness process.

Table 7.3 lists the subjective and objective information which needs to be elicited from the patient presenting with fever.

The answers to the above questions will often lead onto a specific line of examination but it is not a good idea to focus on one isolated symptom or finding. Perform a rapid full examination of the major systems particularly in those who look ill (little sick/big sick).

TIP

Fever associated with persistent vomiting (>12 h) usually requires hospital review

PITFALL

Meningococcal septicaemia can progress rapidly from a patient with minor symptoms to cardiovascular collapse and death within an hour or two[7]

TIP

Jaundice associated with a fever requires hospital admission[3]

Analysis

Fever on its own lasting more than 12 hours with no other associated symptom is fairly rare. It tends either to be due to a mild very short-lived viral insult to the body or to indicate a more significant and often non-infective cause. If you are unsure then further review or more specialist help and investigation is needed.

If a specific cause has been identified from the history and examination then appropriate transfer or treatment should be undertaken according to local protocols and procedures. A raised temperature is usually due to an infection, most commonly viral. The higher the temperature the more likely it is to be bacterial and thus antibiotics to be of benefit. Common causes are infection of the upper or lower respiratory tract, the urinary system and skin. Less common but potentially more serious are infections affecting the central nervous system, the abdomen and septicaemia.

People who have a malignancy are more prone to infections especially if they have recently had chemotherapy and, to a lesser extent, radiotherapy. Patients will usually tell you about this as they are warned to look out for these symptoms by the hospital on discharge from their treatment.

TABLE 7.3 Information that needs to be elicited from the patient presenting with fever

Subjective	Objective
Symptoms How long has the temperature been present? Is it constant or does it fluctuate? Have there been any episodes of 'hot and cold' shivers? Has any medication been taken to help it? If so what was it, how much was taken and how long ago? Did it work? **Associated symptoms** Do they have any pain or swellings anywhere? Are they aware of having a rash? Ask specifically about things such as unsteadiness/vertigo, ability to concentrate, dysuria, frequency, offensive vaginal discharge **Infective contacts/travel** Has anyone else in the family/at work had a similar problem? Has the patient recently returned from abroad? If so where from? Have they been in contact with anyone with a known infectious illness?	**General** Measure vital signs Take the temperature. If the fever seems very mild and the patient reasonably well then the back of your hand applied to the patients forehead in a 'hot/not hot' assessment is acceptable. If the fever seems significant or the patient looks ill then a more objective measurement is mandatory. This may be best provided by an electronic tympanic membrane temperature thermometer though there has been recent debate on their reliability Is there a rash – is it diagnostic of anything? Chickenpox blisters and non-blanching purpuric rashes are generally the only ones to be reliable as indicators of a specific cause Is there muscle tenderness? Is there any evidence of meningism or blunting of consciousness? The latter may be seen in the early stages of encephalitis Check the tympanic membrane, throat and cervical lymph glands Check the eyes for evidence of jaundice **Systems exam** Listen to and percuss the chest Palpate the abdomen and renal angles. Ask the patient to cough – does it hurt their abdomen to do so? This may indicate a degree of peritonism **Tests** Check a urine specimen for blood or nitrites if appropriate – it is always appropriate if no other obvious cause has been found even in the absence of urinary symptoms. This is especially true of the very young and the elderly

Plan

This will depend on a specific cause being found. If no specific diagnosis can be made it is only acceptable to treat the symptom. Antibiotics should certainly not be given to patients without a confirmed cause for their pyrexia as they may mask potentially important future symptoms. The exception would be a patient with suspected septicaemia who is going to be admitted as an emergency.

Paracetamol and ibuprofen may be given according to local protocols in age-related dosages on a regular basis. Check for contraindications such as peptic disease or asthma for ibuprofen. A plan, either patient or practitioner led, should be formulated so that if deterioration occurs or things do not improve within a certain time frame then a review can occur. The well worn advice to parents to tepid sponge or fan their hot child may be helpful in giving them something to do but has minimal effect, if any, over that of appropriate drug therapy.[8]

If a specific diagnosis is made the decision to transfer or treat at home will be based on local procedures, journey times, local resources available for treatment review and the ability of the patient or carer to manage the situation.

Oral antibiotics will be most commonly prescribed but topical preparations (ear drops, nasal ointment, skin cream) can be useful alternatives at times. In some circumstances, and with appropriate local support, people with conditions such as chest and skin infections may be treated with IV antibiotics at home. This requires a 'hospital at home' approach that is becoming more prevalent. Such a service will also provide oxygen, physiotherapy and haematological investigation as required to manage the patient. A blood count, differential white cell count and a CRP can be very useful in deciding what treatment a patient needs and whether or not hospital care is required.[3,9] Significant anaemia, an abnormally high or low white cell count, or a CRP >20 are all indicators of significant disease requiring hospital investigation.

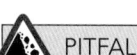

PITFALL

Avoid ibuprofen in asthmatics and those with indigestion symptoms

Communication

Give a clear explanation of the likely diagnosis and the treatment options. Most patients do not want to go to hospital and will usually be very happy with appropriate management that allows them to stay at home.

If there is any uncertainty then the observation of the patient over a short period can be a very important diagnostic tool. This can be arranged either by returning to see the patient or arranging for a more experienced opinion. Communication is vital to the success of such 'wait and see' strategies. Ensure patients and any carers know the treatment plan and how to contact someone urgently if the situation changes.

Nausea, vomiting and fever

Obviously when fever, nausea and vomiting are present together the SOAPC system should be applied in the same way.

| TABLE 7.4 Key points in history and examination (triggers for hospital admission) ||
Nausea/vomiting	Fever
Primary survey positive	Primary survey positive
Pregnancy/pre-existing illness	>39°C
Age <6 months	Associated vomiting
Drug/alcohol ingestion	Associated jaundice
Blood in vomit	Meningism
Severe abdominal pain	Recent travel from a malaria area
Significant dehydration	High (or low) white cell count (if taken)

Subjective and objective

Interestingly the only correlation between fever and severity of illness requiring hospital treatment is the presence of certain other symptoms and signs. One of the most predictive is vomiting. Thus a patient presenting with a high fever (>39°C) and vomiting is highly likely to require hospital admission.[3,5]

Table 7.4 shows the more important features in the history and examination which would point towards the patient requiring hospital admission. Any of the features make admission likely; the presence of any two makes it necessary unless there are local systems allowing a high level of home based investigation and review.

Summary

The vast majority of patients with the symptoms discussed in this chapter will be 'little sick' and will get better with or without treatment. A number of 'little sick' patients will require specific treatment to improve. 'Big sick' patients will be sent to hospital for further investigation and treatment.

Unfortunately a very small number of what appear to be 'little sick' patients rapidly deteriorate and may die. Therefore you must always make sure that someone can call you back if the situation worsens and if necessary give some guidance on what to look for.

If in doubt play safe unless you can arrange a review by a more experienced clinician.

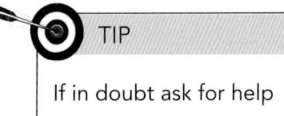

TIP

If in doubt ask for help

References

1 Hodgetts T J, Hall J, Maconochie I, Smart C 1998 The paediatric triage tape. Pre Hospital Immediate Care 2:155–159

2 Woollard M, Jewkes F 2004 Assessment and identification of the paediatric primary survey patients. Emerg Med J 21:511–517

3 Yung A 2000 Approach to undifferentiated fever in adults. In: Cameron P, Jelenik G, Kelly A et al (eds) Textbook of adult emergency medicine. Churchill Livingstone, Edinburgh, p 303–307

4 Armona K, Stephenson T, Macaulb R et al 2001 An evidence and consensus based guideline in acute diarrhoea. Arch Dis Child 85:132–142

5 Knott J C, Tan S L, Street A C, Bailey M, Cameron P 2004 Febrile adults presenting to the emergency department: outcomes and markers of serious illness. Emerg Med J 21:170–174

6 Baraff L J, Bass J W, Fleisher G R et al 1993 Practice guideline for the management of infants and children 0–36 months with fever without source. Ann Emerg Med 22:108–119

7 Jarvis P R E, Wilkinson K N 2004 Meningococcal septicaemia: do not be reassured by normal investigations. Emerg Med J 21:248–249

8 Pursell E 2000 Physical treatment of fever. Arch Dis Child 82:238–239

9 Marco C A, Schoenfeld C N, Hansen K N et al 1995 Fever in geriatric emergency patients: clinical features associated with serious illness. Ann Emerg Med 26:18–24

Further reading

Advanced Life Support Group 2001 Pre-hospital paediatric life support manual. ALSG, Manchester

Hopcroft K, Forte V 1999 Symptom sorter. Radcliffe Medical Press, Oxford

Munro J F, Campbell I W 2000 MacLeod's Clinical examination, 10th edn. Churchill Livingstone, Edinburgh

Robertson-Steel I 2004 'Reforming Emergency Care': the ambulance impact. A personal view. Emerg Med J 21:207–211

Snooks H A, Dale J, Hartley-Sharp C, Halter M 2004 On-scene alternatives for emergency ambulance crews attending patients who do not need to travel to the accident and emergency department: a review of the literature. Emerg Med J 21:212–215

Peter Lawson and Chris Richmond

Problems in older people

Introduction

Medical emergencies are common in older people and they may have difficulty accessing suitable health care once their GP practice is closed. They are less likely to use schemes such as NHS Direct than other parts of the population.[1] They or their carers are more likely to dial 999 if they have an urgent medical problem. The care of the elderly is an increasing proportion of work for GP out-of-hours services, ambulance services and Emergency Departments.

The acute medical problems of older people are often similar to those of younger adults but the presentation can be atypical or there can be a number of co-existing problems that make diagnosis difficult. Further difficulties occur in frailer, older adults who continue to manage at home despite the effects of increasing age and multiple medical problems. In these patients an apparently minor illness can lead to deterioration in a non-specific manner leading to immobility, a fall or acute confusion. The social circumstances and the availability of social support may be of greater importance than the management of the medical illness. Treatment at home is often the preferred and safest option. If a careful clinical and social assessment indicates that the primary problems require social support or nursing expertise, then clinicians must have the option of referring to community support schemes that are now more widely available.

However, major illnesses such as serious infections, heart disease and cancer can also present in a non-specific way. If the presence of one of these conditions is a possibility, then a planned short admission for investigation or early clinic review will be preferable to leaving the patient at home with subsequent admission in a worse condition at a later time.

The management of trauma and surgical emergencies is covered in other chapters. Discussion of single organ emergency problems in older adults such as myocardial infarction will be brief because they should be dealt with in a very similar way to their management in younger adults.

The main emphasis of this chapter is the assessment of physical state, mental state, medication and social circumstances in older adults presenting in a less specific manner such as with general deterioration, falls, confusion and minor injuries.

Community systems for the care of older people

The proper care of the older patient is one of the major priorities of many health systems. Some 'full systems approaches' are emerging but often they lack co-ordination and might only be available for limited times of the week. The bedrock of community care is Primary Care. In the future this will be augmented with support from General Practitioners with a Special Interest in Care of the Elderly or Community Care of the Elderly specialists ('Community Geriatricians') or intensive case management nurses. Acute events are common in this group and there needs to be a co-ordinated system to respond to emergency calls for help.

Figure 8.1 sets out the range of outcomes from community emergency assessment and shows the ideal system to respond to these emergencies.

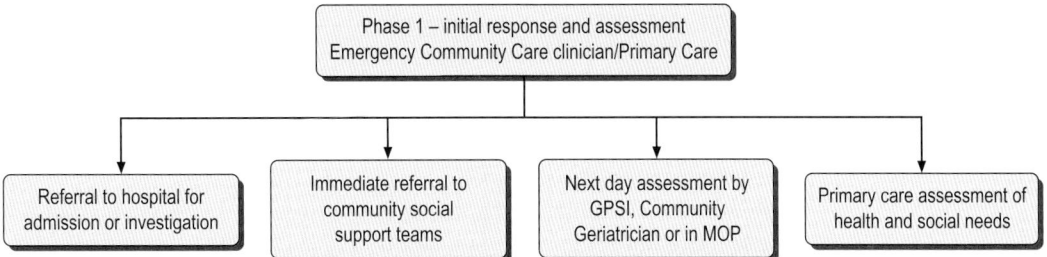

Fig. 8.1 Range of outcomes from community emergency assessment and the ideal system to respond to these emergencies

The community emergency medicine clinician carries out initial crisis support and a brief needs assessment. In significant numbers of older patients this will need to be backed up by either hospital or community services. The keys to success in such a system are excellent communication, mutual respect and clear referral pathways with common documentation systems.

Primary survey positive patients

The criteria for recognition of immediately life threatening problems are the same as for younger patients (Box 8.1). However the interpretation of vital signs may be more difficult and abnormalities need to be taken in context of pre-existing morbidity. A history from a reliable witness is essential. Previous neurological problems can make the GCS permanently <12. Similarly, the elderly are more prone to excessive bradycardia from cardiac medication but on the other hand, symptomatic heart block is common. Oxygen saturations should be interpreted in light of the known medical history and clinical setting.

Primary survey positive patients should be transferred as soon as possible by paramedic ambulance to an A&E Department or an Emergency

---

BOX 8.1 Vital signs indicating 'primary survey positive patient'

- A – potential airway compromise
- unconscious patient/stridor/anaphylaxis/Hx of foreign body
- B – severe distress
- respiratory rate <10 or >29
- oxygen sats <93% on air with no history of COPD
- C – clinical signs of shock
- pulse <50 or >120
- systolic BP <90mmHg
- D – GCS <12 (acute deterioration)
- (acute stroke)

Admissions Unit depending on local protocols. The exception might be those patients with documented 'end of life decisions' such as Advanced Directives and clear, agreed treatment plans which might include 'do not attempt resuscitation' (DNAR) orders.

More than any other group of patients, the older adult might refuse transfer to hospital. If gentle coaxing has failed, carers and family can often be more persuasive. Sometimes it is necessary to consider whether the patient has the mental capacity to refuse transfer for assessment and treatment. In this situation it is possible to agree with family and carers that it is in the patient's best interests to be taken to hospital, especially if they are suffering from serious life-threatening illness. Clear documentation of such decisions is essential in this situation.

Primary survey negative patients

In the elderly patient a greater emphasis must be given to factors other than the 'medical problem' alone. The variables to be considered are given in Box 8.2.

Severity of the medical problem

Patients with signs or symptoms of severe illness should be transferred to hospital unless there are exceptional circumstances. Even with less severe presenting complaints, review in hospital might still be necessary for medical reasons. The elderly are less able to withstand blood loss following, for example, epistaxis or a laceration. They may have a myocardial infarction despite presenting with only minor or no chest pain. There may be only limited signs of peritonism despite significant intra-abdominal pathology. They are at higher risk of developing intracranial haemorrhage and neuropsychological sequelae following a minor head injury. It is best to be cautious and where there is suspicion of serious pathology the patient should be sent to hospital for medical assessment or arrangements made for an immediate visit by the patient's GP. Research has shown that elderly patients with minor falls who dial 999 have a mortality rate of up to 5% at 28 days.

BOX 8.2 **Factors to consider when planning the management of acute events in older people**

- Severity of medical problem
- Cognitive status of the patient
- Social circumstances of the patient
- Availability of community health and social care support

Cognitive status of the patient

The presence of cognitive impairment often renders the history and self-reported ability with activities of daily living unreliable. It is important for any community practitioner to be able to recognise cognitive impairment and, where possible, confirm history with a reliable witness. Impaired cognition in someone living alone might mean they are unable to look after themselves despite an illness being only minor.

Social circumstances

When the medical condition does not of itself indicate that hospital admission is required, the patient's social circumstances may have a large bearing on whether they can remain at home. The availability of someone to provide food and hydration, give medication and call for help if their condition deteriorates is crucial for a person who has had a fall with soft tissue injury, has a chest infection or a minor head injury. If the patient is living alone, explore other sources of help such as family or friends. If such help is not available then it might be necessary to arrange emergency support from community rapid response teams.

A further complication is that the patient may be the main carer for someone else. If this is the case, social services should be contacted to arrange a sitting service or temporary respite placement until the carer is able to resume those duties. A review of social circumstances includes finding out if the patient has someone who could act as a carer or if they provide care for someone themselves.

> **TIP**
>
> The patient may be the main carer for a partner or spouse; if they are admitted to hospital you may need to arrange care for the other person

Health and social care services

Across the UK there are a range of services under a variety of names with the primary purpose of supporting older patients at home or within supported settings outside hospital. Knowledge of the locally available services and how to contact them is crucial. Most services provided at home include care workers, nurses and therapists. A relatively new concept is that of 'intensive case management' – patients with high medical, nursing or social needs may have specialist teams already assigned to their care.

Non-specific presentations of illness in older patients

Patients presenting with non-specific complaints make up a large proportion of most hospitals' acute medical admissions. The presentation can be with confusion, falls, being 'off legs' or with the label of being 'a social admission'.

These 'non-specific' presentations are common and create significant diagnostic and management problems. A seemingly minor injury or illness can be due to several underlying medical conditions. The commonest causes of 'non-specific' presentations are listed in Box 8.3. Full details are listed in many textbooks.[2] The presenting complaint may be determined more by pre-existing mental or physical frailty than the acute illness.

The rest of this chapter will address the management of these patients by emergency community care clinicians or GPs. This will include taking a history, performing a focused physical and mental status examination and formulating a management plan.

BOX 8.3 A brief summary of causes of falls and acute confusion

- Medications, e.g. sedatives, hypotensive agents
- Infection, e.g. chest and urinary tract
- Metabolic disturbance, e.g. dehydration, alcohol, low sodium or low glucose
- Neurological event or conditions, e.g. TIA, seizure
- Cardiovascular event or conditions, e.g. causing low cerebral perfusion
- Environmental causes, e.g. unfamiliar surroundings

Subjective information – history

Not all patients in this age group are able to give a reliable history and thus it is essential to glean as much information as possible from carers. Details of general history taking are reviewed in Chapter 2. Specific elements of the history, including the social history and features highlighted in Box 8.2, will determine the need for further investigation or transfer.

Objective information – examination

Vital signs (Box 8.4) are, as always, important but may be altered by pre-existing morbidity. The GCS is the most obvious example where pre-existing confusion will make assessment of the verbal score difficult. Similarly, pulse and blood pressure may be altered by pre-existing medications such as β-blockers. Any concern about the vital signs or general appearance of the patient should trigger an immediate hospital assessment.

The next stage is a *focused systems examination*. A full examination is required but given the huge number of problems causing falls or confusion certain areas should be given additional emphasis. The examination described in Box 8.5 is aimed at patients with falls but most also applies to patients with confusion, including assessments of both physical and mental status.

BOX 8.4 Assessment of vital signs and general appearance

Vital signs
■ pulse
■ blood pressure
■ respiratory rate
■ oxygen saturations
■ temperature
■ GCS

General
■ does the patient appear unwell?
■ colour, rash, sweating
■ hydration, eyes, mouth

BOX 8.5 Examination and simple tests for older patients with immobility, falls or acute confusion

General appearance
■ Evidence of not coping at home
■ Parkinsonian features, e.g. rigidity, tremor
■ Depression
■ Thyroid status
■ Flushed, pyrexial

Cardiovascular
■ Pulse including peripheral pulses
■ Lying and standing blood pressure
■ Source of emboli – heart rhythm, murmurs and bruits

Neuromuscular system
■ Lateralising signs
■ Parkinson's disease
■ Proximal muscle weakness
■ Gait – 'Get up and Go' test[3]

Abdomen
■ Masses and constipation

Infection
■ Chest auscultation
■ Urine dipstick

Mental test score
■ Hodkinson AMT[4] (see Box 8.6)

Tests
■ 12-lead ECG
■ BM stix
■ Urine dipstick

There are many tools available for the assessment of cognitive function. Each has limitations but they can give an indication of problems with cognition and can be used to follow progress. Box 8.6 shows the 10-question Hodkinson Abbreviated Mental Test score which combines brevity with validity. Questions have to be asked in the order shown and are given 1 mark for the correct answer or no mark. A score below 8 out of 10 implies cognitive impairment.

BOX 8.6 10 question Hodkinson AMT (see Hodkinson[4] for correct use)

1. Age (to the exact year)
2. Time (to the nearest hour)
3. Address for recall at end of test – this should be repeated by the patient to ensure it has been heard correctly: 42 West Street
4. Year (exactly)
5. Name of place
6. Recognition of two people
7. Date of birth (day and month needed exactly)
8. Year of First World War (either year of start or finish)
9. Name of present monarch
10. Count backwards from 20 to 1 (immediate spontaneous corrections are allowed)
3a. Ask for recall of the given address

Tests

Examination of a 12-lead electrocardiograph (ECG) is important if there is concern about a silent myocardial infarction. However, it should be remembered that it can often be normal in someone with unstable or a new presentation of angina – these patients should be transferred to the Emergency Department for assessment. In someone who has lost consciousness without palpitations, chest pain, seizure or injury and has fully recovered, a normal 12-lead ECG means transfer to A&E is not routinely necessary.

Blood glucose measurement should be routine in anyone with a history of diabetes or presenting with increasing confusion or blackouts.

Urine dipstick testing should be performed for anyone with symptoms of a urinary tract infection, such as the recent onset of confusion or signs of sepsis. Urinary tract infections affect a significant proportion of older adults.

Management plan

Older adults prefer to be treated at home and where possible this should be facilitated. Removal to unfamiliar environments can precipitate distress and confusion and lead to a further deterioration in the patient's clinical condition and a further loss of independence. Transfer to hospital must therefore be reserved for those cases where further investigations are likely to be of benefit or where an adequate standard of care cannot be provided in the home. Competent elderly patients must be fully involved in making decisions about their care plan and any interventions must always be subject to their fully informed consent. Different management strategies are now discussed.

Treat and leave/review

Details of treatment of specific minor injuries are described in Chapter 13. Patients with minor illness can be treated at home if adequate support is available. However, it should be ensured that the patient and their carers clearly understand when and how to seek further advice or help if their condition does not improve or deteriorates. If patients do not require further referral their GP must still be informed of the 'emergency' episode and they can then decide when to review the patient.

Examples of treat and leave patients include those with chronic balance and gait problems despite support from the falls service, those with an obvious minor infection suitable for treatment with oral antibiotics, or those with soft tissue injury but no bony tenderness and requiring only simple analgesia.

Treat and refer

Many emergency calls reveal increased social care or community nursing needs. The occurrence of a previously un-investigated, non-specific presentation of illness in an older person also highlights the need for referral for a specialist assessment that can be started in Primary Care. Most health communities now have care pathways for dealing with patients presenting in a variety of ways – for example, following a fall. Those involved in emergency care must know how to access these pathways of care and how to obtain rapid response nursing and social care.

Another example suitable for treat and refer might be a patient who has fallen with a brief loss of consciousness or short period of palpitations. If they have recovered and have a normal 12-lead ECG they may be suitable to be left at home but referred for urgent review in a hospital or community clinic. An abnormal 12-lead ECG in the patient with loss of consciousness would, however, require hospital assessment.

Another reason for referral to hospital would be for X-rays to exclude fracture. Referral pathways should be established to enable the community emergency practitioner to directly refer patients for an appropriate X-ray with varying urgency. X-ray of what might be a minor fracture may be deferred if pain can be controlled with simple analgesics to avoid an admission in the middle of the night. However, if the patient is unable to care for themselves or the suspected fracture is associated with significant pain or neurovascular problems, an X-ray may be required in a shorter time-scale. Self-mobilising patients with suspected bony injuries to the upper limbs will rarely require transfer by emergency ambulance and alternative forms of transport should be considered.

Treat and transfer

There are several groups of patients in this category. Some have worrying symptoms, as in Box 8.7. Others are less ill but lack suitable support at home or appropriate services to support the patient at home cannot be organised. If a bed in an Intermediate Care facility cannot be arranged, these patients will need to be taken to hospital. Finally, there are those who cannot be properly assessed at home and who need to be brought to the Emergency Department for this to be done.

When transfer is required, the community emergency practitioner can make an important contribution to the work of the ambulance service by recommending the most appropriate form of transport for patients requiring admission. For example, a patient requiring no care other than assistance to get to the vehicle will not require a paramedic staffed emergency ambulance, and can be safely cared for by staff with more limited training, thus preserving scarce resources for those patients most likely to benefit from them.

Other factors to consider

Any clinician seeing an older person in their home has the opportunity to assess the level of care that person is receiving and whether they are being

---

BOX 8.7 Worrying features making hospital referral more likely

Falls
- Recurrent blackouts
- Altered behaviour before or after a fall
- Associated symptoms, e.g.
  - ischaemic chest pain requiring repeat ECG or cardiac enzymes
  - 'dizziness' with a postural BP drop or with vertigo
- New drowsiness
- Inability to bear weight or use arms due to pain
- Hip pain

Confusion
- Acute onset
- Recent medication changes
- New symptoms such as personality change or focal weakness
- Recent head injury
- Behaviour likely to lead to harm for self or others

subject to abuse. The pattern of injury seen in physical abuse is often similar to those sustained during a fall but if the patient denies a fall the possibility of elder abuse should be considered. It should also be remembered that psychological, financial and sexual abuse plus abuse through neglect can all lead to physical and mental decline resulting in an emergency assessment. If elder abuse is suspected, social services should be informed. Please visit www.elderabuse.org.uk for more information and advice.

Summary

Practitioners dealing with emergencies in older adults in the community must be able to recognise the atypical presentation of illness in older people and have a high index of suspicion that apparently innocent symptoms can be the presentation of serious underlying pathology. It must also be remembered that the common medical emergencies of younger adults generally occur more frequently in older adults and require similar treatment.

Necessary skills include clear communication with patients although on occasions witnesses must be used to obtain relevant information. A focused examination including a mental state test is often necessary when dealing with non-specific illness in the older patient and when determining if someone can be left at home.

A home visit allows assessment of the patient's social circumstances and emergency practitioners might sometimes need to make adjustments to ensure the safety of the patient in their surroundings if they are to be left at home or subject to a delay in transfer. Evidence of neglect by the patient or by others should also be looked for when attending the patient at home. The combination of social and medical assessment, linked to knowledge of the services available locally will determine where the patient's care will be best delivered.

With an older patient it is safer to err on the side of caution to avoid denying patients a specialist assessment. For many this will need to be a comprehensive geriatric assessment performed after the emergency episode has passed.

References

1   NHS Direct in England 2002 Report by the Comptroller and Auditor General. National Audit Office, London
2   Kenny R A 2000 Falls and syncope. In: Evans G J, Williams F T, Beattie L B, Michel J-P, Wilcock GK (eds) Oxford textbook of geriatric medicine. Oxford University Press, Oxford, p 111–124
3   Mathias S, Nayak U S, Isaacs B 1986 Balance in elderly patients: The 'get-up and go' test. Arch Phys Med Rehabil 67:387–389
4   Hodkinson H M 1972 Evaluation of a mental test score for assessment of mental impairment in the elderly. Age Ageing 1:233–238

James Gray, Jim Wardrope and Diana Jane Fothergill

Abdominal pain, abdominal pain in women, complications of pregnancy and labour

Introduction

Large numbers of patients with abdominal pain present to their GPs and Emergency Departments every year. The majority requires no specific medical intervention but some will require urgent hospital admission. The elderly and paediatric patient present particular challenges. The very young often give a poor history or can very quickly deteriorate.

BOX 9.1 Chapter objectives

- Recognise the severely ill patient and manage appropriately
- Evaluate and manage stable patients
- Management of abdominal pain in women
- Management of pregnancy and its complications

BOX 9.2 Key points in assessing abdominal pain

- Abdominal pain is very common
- The very young and very old can present a specific challenge
- It is often unnecessary to make a diagnosis in order to plan your management
- In women of childbearing age always consider the possibility of pregnancy

---

The elderly may have a very complicated medical history and misleading signs. A longitudinal study found that 50% of elderly patients (65 or over) with abdominal pain required admission.[1] Due to the difficulty of assessment in these groups of patients you should have a lower threshold for referral.

Abdominal pain has numerous causes but it is not necessary to reach a specific diagnosis. The aim is to decide on a management plan, to know when to monitor a patient at home and to rule out the more serious pathology. Most patients can be adequately assessed by the simple techniques described and an accurate plan formed for the patient's further management.

This chapter will focus on initial assessment and management and not on specific conditions (Boxes 9.1 and 9.2). There are numerous texts which will give the basic outline of symptoms for different pathologies.[2,3] More than 30 women die each year in the UK as a direct consequence of pregnancy. The Confidential Enquiry into Maternal Deaths 1997–99[4] stated that 'Women are still dying of potentially treatable conditions where the use of simple diagnostic guidelines may help to identify conditions such as ectopic pregnancy, sepsis and pulmonary embolism'.

The primary survey

All patients should be assessed using the ABCDE approach. Abdominal pain can be immediately life threatening (primary survey positive). Such cases need to be identified early so that appropriate care can start immediately (Box 9.3).

> **BOX 9.3 Life-threatening causes of abdominal pain**
>
> - Generalised peritonitis with shock
> - Acute bowel obstruction
> - Ruptured abdominal aortic aneurysm
> - Acute mesenteric infarction
> - Ruptured ectopic pregnancy
> - Placental abruption and other complications of pregnancy
> - Toxic shock syndrome

TIP

Do not lie a heavily pregnant woman on her back

The unusual cause of shock-like syndrome in pregnancy is supine hypotension. If a pregnant woman is laid on her back for a prolonged period the uterus obstructs the inferior vena cava resulting in a drop in venous return, cardiac output and hypotension. If the uterus is palpable above the umbilicus, lie the patient in the left lateral position.

Primary survey positive

These patients present in a variety of ways but airway and breathing assessment requires the same approach as in any other life-threatening situation. Shock is the main immediately life-threatening problem in patients with abdominal pain (Box 9.4).

Shock can be due to either hypovolaemia or sepsis. On route to hospital obtain IV access and draw blood for cross-matching. Remember to complete the patient details on the blood specimen tube. No intervention should delay transfer to definitive medical care. IV fluid resuscitation in abdominal haemorrhage should be based on the principle of *hypotensive resuscitation*, aiming to give enough fluid to maintain a radial pulse.[4]

TIP

If the radial pulse is palpable, the blood pressure can be assumed to be adequate. If absent, aim to give fluid until radial pulse is palpable again

These patients are likely to be in pain. IV opiate analgesia may be given en route but monitor the BP closely and titrate small doses in unstable patients. Evidence shows that pain relief does not affect subsequent clinical assessment and that it removes damaging physiological stresses and improves accuracy of examination[5] (Box 9.5).

The most common life-threatening problems are summarised in Box 9.3. However many common abdominal problems such as acute appendicitis can be life-threatening if not promptly diagnosed and treated. This emphasises the importance of reassessment of patients with continuing or worsening symptoms.

> **BOX 9.4 Common presentations of 'primary survey positive' patients**
>
> - Collapse
> - Shock
> - Rigid abdomen
> - Heavy vaginal bleeding
> - Complications of labour

BOX 9.5 Key points in treating 'primary survey positive' patients

- Some causes of abdominal pain are immediately life-threatening
- Treat as able but do not delay definitive transfer
- Fluids should be given based upon the principle of hypotensive resuscitation
- Intravenous opiate analgesia can be given to relieve pain

Consider potentially serious medical conditions not directly related to the gastrointestinal tract that can also present as abdominal pain (Box 9.6). A focused history and examination will help in identifying such cases (see below). Specific potential threats to life in women are shown in Box 9.7.

Ectopic pregnancy classically presents with vaginal bleeding and abdominal pain, but there may also be associated internal bleeding which may give rise to shoulder tip pain. The degree of shock may be disproportional to the observed blood loss. The woman may be unaware of pregnancy and may not give a history of a missed period. These patients need fast transport to an appropriate unit. Obtain venous access en route if possible. Give enough fluids to maintain the radial pulse and high flow oxygen. Alert the receiving unit and ensure the gynaecologist is aware.

An incomplete miscarriage may result in products of conception caught in the cervix which leads to profound vagal stimulation with bradycardia and shock. These patients need urgent hospital admission because removal of these products will lead to a rapid clinical improvement and reduction in bleeding. Any tissue passed should accompany the woman to hospital.

Pulmonary embolism is still responsible for a number of maternal deaths. Have a low index of suspicion and refer pregnant women with shortness of breath or pleuritic chest pain.

BOX 9.6 Medical conditions presenting with abdominal pain

- Inferior myocardial infarction
- Pneumonia
- Pulmonary infarction
- Diabetic ketoacidosis
- Inflammatory bowel disease
- Pyelonephritis

BOX 9.7 Potential threats to life in women

- Ectopic pregnancy
- Incomplete miscarriage
- Genital tract trauma
- Pulmonary embolism
- Toxic shock syndrome

Toxic shock syndrome is caused by invasive staphylococcal or streptococcal infections and is usually associated with tampon use. The picture is one of septicaemic shock. Manage by fast transport, IV access en route and oxygen.

Problems in later pregnancy

A number of complications of pregnancy pose potential threats to life, not only for the mother but also to the fetus (Box 9.8). This is a very high risk area of practice where the inexperienced practitioner must ask for the patient to be reviewed by the obstetric team.

BOX 9.8 Potential threats to life in late pregnancy

- Placental abruption
- Placenta praevia
- Pregnancy-induced hypertension (pre-eclampsia and eclampsia)
- Pulmonary embolism

Placental abruption

This occurs when the placenta separates from the uterus prior to birth. There is constant severe pain, and the uterus usually will be rigid and with a sustained contraction. There may be vaginal bleeding but much of the blood is retained within the uterus so the degree of shock will usually be out of proportion to the amount of revealed bleeding. Rapid transfer to hospital is essential – with IV access and high flow oxygen. The receiving unit should be alerted as emergency caesarean section will probably be required.

Placenta praevia

This often presents with painless vaginal bleeding unless the patient is in labour. It is due to the placenta covering the internal part of the cervix. This can lead to catastrophic vaginal bleeding as the cervix dilates at the start of labour.

Pregnancy induced hypertension – pre-eclampsia and eclampsia

In early pregnancy the blood pressure is usually lower than normal. A blood pressure of 140/90 mmHg might seem fairly normal but in a pregnant woman implies pregnancy-induced hypertension until proven otherwise.

Pre-eclampsia is a condition specifically associated with pregnancy, usually but not always occurring in the late stages of pregnancy. Classically it presents with hypertension, proteinuria and oedema (Box 9.9). When the condition worsens the woman may complain of upper right sided

> **BOX 9.9 Symptoms and signs of severe pre-eclampsia**
>
> - Headache
> - Visual disturbance
> - Upper abdominal pain
> - Generalised oedema
> - Brisk reflexes
> - Reduced urine output
> - Blood pressure >140/90 or rise in diastolic from previous readings
> - Ankle swelling
> - Proteinuria

or epigastric abdominal pain, headache, nausea and vomiting. She may become confused and have very brisk reflexes. Fitting can then follow. Unless the woman is a known epileptic, any fit in pregnancy is managed as a probable eclamptic fit. Fits due to eclampsia may pose significant airway problems. Manage these as in any other fit by simple airway manoeuvres. If the fit is not self-limiting intravenous diazemuls should be given supplemented by magnesium sulphate once the patient arrives in hospital. It is also essential to control the blood pressure as soon as possible. Urgent transfer to an obstetric unit is required.

Evaluation of the stable patient

If the primary survey shows no requirement for resuscitation then a secondary survey can be undertaken using the SOAPC system. History and examination has been shown to be very effective in distinguishing organic and non-organic causes of pain.[6]

Subjective information

The history is the most important aid in reaching a diagnosis. The correct questions can very quickly allow the assessor to gauge the severity of the problem as well rule out the serious causes of abdominal pain. The main questions are related to the pain (Box 9.10), other symptoms, previous treatment or medical contacts in this episode, as well as the standard past medical, drug, allergy and social history.

Pain

Onset
Pain with a sudden onset is likely to be an acute severe event, e.g. ruptured aneurysm or perforated viscus. In contrast a gradual onset suggests an inflammatory or infective cause.

BOX 9.10 Questions that should be asked about the pain: 'OPQRST'

- Onset
- Provoking or palliative factors
- Quality – constant/colicky
- Radiation and site of pain, e.g. shoulder tip
- Severity and systemic symptoms
- Timing – was onset sudden or insidious, did it change over time?

Precipitating and palliative factors – quality, timing and radiation

Precipitating and palliative factors may give important clues. The patient with peritonitis will usually lie still with movement or coughing worsening the pain. In contrast the patient with colic will often be restless, trying to find a comfortable position.

Quality Abdominal pain is commonly described as 'peritoneal' or 'colicky'. If the parietal peritoneum is aggravated then the pain will be well localised to the area of the pathology. In contrast, visceral pain tends to be poorly localised and based on the embryonic divisions of foregut (mouth to proximal half of the duodenum), midgut (distal half of the duodenum to middle of the transverse colon), and hindgut (rest of colon to rectum). Pain from foregut structures is referred to the upper abdomen, from midgut around the umbilicus, hindgut, and lower abdomen.

Colicky pain is usually due to spasm of a tubular structure, often around a blockage. Colicky pain is therefore more commonly biliary, intestinal or ureteric in origin.

Radiation of the pain may assist in diagnosis. Renal pain tends to radiate 'loin to groin'. Diaphragmatic irritation, e.g. ruptured ectopic, may radiate to the shoulder tip due to their common innervation (C3,4,5).

Systemic symptoms (nausea/vomiting/urinary/gynaecological) may be helpful in diagnosis but can also be misleading. For example, constipation is associated with obstruction but is not always present. It is important to establish the patient's normal bowel habit.

Diarrhoea is normal in gastroenteritis but may also be due to overflow related to chronic constipation, irritation of the pelvic peritoneum (e.g. pelvic appendicitis) or partial obstruction. Faecal blood may indicate inflammatory bowel disease, cancer or parasitic infection.

Urinary symptoms may suggest urinary tract infection (UTI) but not all UTIs cause abdominal pain.

In the female patient a menstrual history should be taken. Gynaecological causes should be considered. *All women of childbearing age with abdominal pain who have missed a period must have ectopic pregnancy excluded.*

Timing Pain may change over time, e.g. appendicitis starts with a colicky periumbilical pain due to obstruction. This then leads to infection and a localised inflammation of the parietal peritoneum. Is the pain related to food, passing urine or faeces?

Previous history

If the patient has previously presented with the same problem it is important to keep an open mind. Diseases can progress, complications may arise and the patient's condition change.

Past medical history (Box 9.11) can reveal other abdominal problems or chronic illnesses (e.g. angina) which may point you towards a diagnosis.

Certain drugs are associated with gastrointestinal side effects. Non-steroidal anti-inflammatory agents increase risk of peptic ulceration and bleeding. Many antibiotics cause diarrhoea and some can cause life-threatening problems such as pseudomembranous colitis.

BOX 9.11 Key points in taking the history

- A good history is your most important diagnostic tool
- Always repeat a full history even if the patient has been seen previously
- Do not forget gynaecological problems in the female patient

---

Objective information

This consists of examination and investigations on scene (if available or relevant) and is summarised in Box 9.12.

BOX 9.12 Summary scheme of examination of patient with abdominal pain

General
- Posture – curled up/agitated (colic); flat/bent knees (peritonism)
- Colour – pale; jaundice
- Vital signs
- Mouth (fetor), tongue, skin turgor for hydration
- Lymph nodes

Abdomen
- *Look* – distension, movement, flanks bruising
- *Feel* – evidence of peritonitis, pulses, hernial orifices
- *Listen* – bowel sounds
- Testicles
- PR/PV if appropriate (be cautious if no chaperone)

Other
- Respiratory system
- Cardiovascular system

Patient preparation

In an ideal setting, examination of the abdomen would involve ensuring that the patient is exposed from 'nipple to knee', and PR or PV examinations performed (Box 9.13). However it is very likely that these will be difficult and often impossible in the community setting. If carrying out a PR/PV examination, explain all stages to the patient and have a chaperone present at all times. Exceptions to this rule would be where the patient is very unwell and there is an obvious clinical need, for example heavy PV bleeding or imminent childbirth.

BOX 9.13 Key points in the examination

■ Examination helps to refine your history diagnosis
■ A structured examination will help avoid missing important information
■ Do not forget the hernial orifices
■ PR and PV should only be done if adding useful clinical information which may prevent hospital referral
■ Consider near patient testing in selected cases

Vital signs

Vital signs have been discussed in primary survey and are often the most sensitive indicators of a serious problem. It is unlikely that the normotensive, apyrexial patient with a pulse rate of 80 has an immediately life-threatening abdominal problem at the time of examination, but is no guarantee that such a condition may not develop.

Other general signs such as assessment of hydration and smelling the breath for fetor (sweet smell indicating ketosis) may help assess the general state of health.

The abdomen

The patient should be fully exposed within the boundaries of decency and careful inspection carried out.

Look

Look especially for obvious distension, swellings, herniae, or other masses or scars of previous operations. The patient should be examined with the arms by the side so as to decrease abdominal wall muscle tension.

Ask the patient to take a deep breath and then to cough while observing the patient's reaction and abdominal movement. The patient with peritoneal irritation will avoid movement or the pain will be increased.

Feel

Before palpating the abdomen ask the patient to point to the site of greatest pain and then commence examination as far away from this point as possible. Initially use gentle, shallow palpation before palpating more deeply. In an area of specific tenderness due to peritoneal irritation there will usually be guarding – a spasm of the overlying abdominal muscles.

Percussion over the area of tenderness giving pain suggests peritoneal irritation. Testing for rebound tenderness is no longer considered appropriate.

Assess for organomegaly of the liver and spleen by always starting in the right lower quadrant and moving toward the hypochondrium to avoid missing a grossly enlarged organ.

Murphy's sign is elicited by pressing the fingertips up towards the right costal margin and asking the patient to breathe deeply. If the gallbladder is inflamed, the patient will experience pain when breathing in as the gallbladder descends and comes into contact with the palpating hand.

Always assess the inguinal and femoral hernial orifices. Obstruction secondary to a strangulated or incarcerated hernia is a diagnosis often missed by inexperienced clinicians. It is usually appropriate at this point to assess the scrotum in the male.

Listen

Auscultate for at least 1 minute in a single location. Absence of bowel sounds suggests significant pathology whilst high pitched tinkling sounds may also suggest obstruction.

Rectal and vaginal exam

In the community setting these examinations may be difficult. Always ensure you have a chaperone present if you undertake these examinations. Unless they are likely to add useful diagnostic information that might prevent hospital referral, they should be omitted.

Abdominal examination is difficult in overweight, elderly and paediatric patients, and those with a reduced conscious level. You need to take into account the less than ideal nature of your examination in the analysis of the problem.

Investigations

Investigations that may be of use in the community are urine dipstick testing for urinary tract infection or haematuria, blood glucose testing in possible diabetic keto-acidosis, and a pregnancy test in any woman of childbearing age. This should be performed with patient consent. In atypical epigastric pain an ECG may be indicated.

Analysis

Certain symptoms are absolute indications for admission whilst others are more relative and rely on assessment and the degree of certainty about the diagnosis (Table 9.1). In the woman of child-bearing age, always consider the possibility of ectopic pregnancy. If there is any doubt, discussion with the gynaecology team is mandatory. Table 9.2 lists the common diagnoses in patients with acute abdominal pain and the 'classical' signs and symptoms. However many abdominal conditions can present in an atypical fashion, also signs and symptoms may change; thus the need for a high index of suspicion.

TABLE 9.1 Absolute and relative indications for referral to hospital

Absolute	Relative
Primary survey positive	Uncertain diagnosis
Peritonitis	Poor social circumstances/no supervision
Vital signs abnormal	Pyrexia of unknown origin
Definite diagnosis requiring admission	Very young
Signs of obstruction	Very elderly
Suspected abdominal aortic aneurysm	Pregnancy
Unwell patient	
Opiate analgesia required	

Abdominal pain in women

The assessment principles are described above. The menstrual history must be taken and pregnancy or its complications always suspected (Box 9.14).

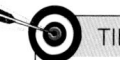 TIP

Always consider the possibility of ectopic pregnancy in women with abdominal pain. If no history of missed period, check if last period was normal (in time, duration and blood loss). Ask about contraception

Ectopic pregnancy

This is a diagnosis which should be considered in all women of reproductive age. Classically the patient will have lower abdominal pain, a history of a late or missed period and signs of peritoneal irritation. Unfortunately the symptoms and signs may be misleading. You should have a high index of suspicion if the woman has a history of infertility, has missed a period whilst using an intrauterine contraceptive device, or has been sterilised. The management is outlined above.

TABLE 9.2 Common diagnoses and their common presentation	
Diagnosis	Presentation
Non-specific abdominal pain	Usually vague history of symptoms with non-specific triggers. Little to find on examination. Usually self-limiting. If pain continues/worsens consider other diagnoses
Gastroenteritis	Usually history of eating possible contaminated food/contact with other cases. Diarrhoea and vomiting classical. Usually self-limiting
Appendicitis	Typically initial central vague pain that becomes localised to the right iliac fossa. Often associated with vomiting and anorexia
Leaking aneurysm	If acute rupture often sudden acute 'tearing' pain or collapse. Pain radiates through to the back or groin, often with a palpable pulsating midline abdominal mass. May have history of known aneurysm
Peptic ulcer	Usually upper abdominal pain associated with eating. Perforation gives severe pain often through to back and peritonitis
Biliary colic and acute cholecystitis	Colicky right upper quadrant pain or epigastric pain often radiating to the back. In acute cholecystitis may be toxic and pyrexial with tenderness (Murphy's sign)
Acute pancreatitis	Often sudden onset of severe peritoneal pain in the upper abdomen, with signs of shock
Acute intestinal obstruction	Classically constipation and vomiting. In a more proximal obstruction vomiting is the main symptom. There may be significant fluid and electrolyte losses
Renal colic	Usually sudden onset severe colicky pain in the loin with radiation to groin. Voltarol PO or PR is an effective analgesic. Beware of this diagnosis in the elderly. Patients with abdominal aortic aneurysm often have haematuria
Small bowel infarction	Acute, severe abdominal pain in the elderly, out of proportion to clinical signs often around RIF. Rapidly become hypovolaemic and shocked. May have history of colicky post-prandial abdominal pain or of atrial fibrillation

---

BOX 9.14 Important causes of abdominal pain in women

- *Common*
    - Urinary tract infection
    - Pelvic inflammatory disease
    - Dysmenorrhoea
    - Labour
- *Less common*
    - Ectopic pregnancy
    - Appendicitis
    - Biliary colic
    - Ovarian syndromes
    - Miscarriage
- *Uncommon*
    - Ovarian hyperstimulation syndrome
    - Curtis–Fitzhugh syndrome
    - Toxic shock syndrome

Common problems

Cystitis

Cystitis is very common with classical symptoms of frequency and dysuria. Systemic symptoms such as nausea, vomiting and fever are not usual in simple cystitis. The abdominal pain is less of a feature than the urinary symptoms and the abdomen is rarely tender. Urinalysis gives a typical picture with protein and white cells and often some blood. One major pitfall is that other causes of pelvic inflammation can also cause frequency and dysuria. For example a pelvic appendicitis will cause abdominal pain, dysuria, frequency and even protein, blood and white cells on urinalysis.

Most women with cystitis will be systemically well and will have no major abdominal signs. Cystitis is diagnosed by sending a midstream specimen of urine for culture and sensitivity and is treated with oral fluids and antibiotics. Alkylating agents may give symptomatic relief.

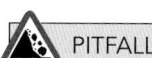

PITFALL

Any cause of pelvic inflammation may cause dysuria and frequency

Pyelonephritis

Pyelonephritis is associated with urinary symptoms but the patient is unwell, has loin pain, is pyrexial, and often has nausea or vomiting. If the systemic symptoms are mild then outpatient treatment is possible. If the patient cannot tolerate oral antibiotics or has significant systemic symptoms and signs then they will need referral to hospital.

Dysmenorrhoea

Pain at the time of the period is an extremely common symptom. If the period is late or the amount of bleeding is abnormal then ectopic pregnancy or miscarriage should be considered. There are no major abdominal signs. A pregnancy test should be done. A NSAID such as mefenamic acid is the best symptomatic treatment for this problem.

Early pregnancy vaginal bleeding/miscarriage

A miscarriage is the loss of a pregnancy before 20 weeks gestation. The usual symptom is vaginal bleeding. There is often some abdominal pain but this is not usually severe. If the bleeding is not severe (for example less than in a normal period), the pregnancy is less than 12 weeks and the patient is well and stable, contact the gynaecology unit to arrange review at an early pregnancy assessment unit. If the bleeding is heavy, there is tachycardia or bradycardia and hypotension, products of conception have been passed or if the abdominal pain is severe, refer for immediate gynaecological assessment.

Pelvic inflammatory disease

Infections of the fallopian tubes and surrounding tissues are common in sexually active women. Typically there is a history of vaginal discharge and lower abdominal pain. The differential diagnosis includes urinary tract infection, appendicitis and ectopic pregnancy. Patients with mild symptoms should be advised to consult their primary care doctor or go to a genitourinary medicine clinic as soon as possible. Patients who have missed a period, have a positive pregnancy test or have significant systemic upset should be referred to hospital for further investigations.

Ovarian cysts, mid-cycle ovulation pain

Ovarian cysts may rupture or undergo torsion. The cyst may not be large enough to feel abdominally but there will be rebound tenderness and signs of peritonism. There may be a mild pyrexia. If the right ovary is involved the presentation is similar to appendicitis. Refer to the gynaecology team.

Mid-cycle ovulation pain occurs at ovulation. As the follicle ruptures there may be mild irritation of the peritoneum. The patient is well, she is at the mid-point of a normal menstrual cycle, the symptoms are short lived, vital signs are normal, there are no systemic symptoms. Check a pregnancy test. Advise simple analgesia but emphasise the need to seek further advice if the pain does not settle, gets worse or other symptoms develop.

Ovarian hyperstimulation syndrome This is a gynaecological emergency, which may be life-threatening. It generally occurs in women who are having ovulation induced under the care of an assisted conception unit. Large cysts appear in the ovaries and fluid shifts from the circulation to produce ascites and a shock-like clinical syndrome. These patients will have abdominal pain and significant systemic upset. If a woman undergoing IVF or other methods of assisted conception develops abdominal pain, refer urgently to the appropriate gynaecological team.

Plan for patients with abdominal pain

A risk stratification approach will give a good guide as to the appropriate management plan. This involves using your analysis to put patients in one of five groups:

- Group 1 – Features suggesting hospital referral. There are very clear signs of definite surgical pathology with a large number of typical features of disease, for example classical appendicitis. In these patients the management plan is straightforward and little further investigation is needed in the emergency department. These patients should, therefore, be referred to the appropriate inpatient team (e.g. surgical admissions unit).
- Group 2 – Patients who need a disease 'rule-out'. There are borderline cases with some features of a diagnosis but the clinical picture is not sufficiently clear to make a definite decision on management. They need further investigation and possibly further

observation. This group will include the very young, the older patient and cases where there are communication difficulties. These may need to be referred to A&E or to the appropriate inpatient team.

- Group 3 – Common features allowing diagnosis of a problem which may be treated at home. For example the young woman with definite signs of urinary tract infection and no signs of other pathology, or a clear history of a likely self-limiting gastroenteritis in an otherwise fit and healthy person.
- Group 4 – Type of patient who may be treated by a wait-and-see approach. This group has no specific symptoms or signs that indicate serious pathology at the time of assessment. Do not give a 'diagnosis' such as 'constipation' or 'UTI' when there are no specific symptoms or signs or confirmatory test results. These patients may be managed at home with advice that the diagnosis is not clear but *at present* there are no signs of serious pathology. The patient should be advised to seek further advice if symptoms fail to settle or get worse.
- Group 5 – Social implications. Some patients may need referral, such as the very elderly or very young, due to difficulty coping at home, as well as the tendency for more rapid deterioration in condition.

> ◎ TIP
>
> As a general principle, if a patient consults for a third time in a few days with the same problem then they should be referred for a specialist opinion

Communication

Communication in abdominal pain is both with the patient and with other agencies.

The patient

If the patient is to be managed at home then give a full explanation of your findings and, if possible, likely diagnosis and its usual progression/resolution. If the diagnosis remains unclear reassure the patient that there are no signs of serious illness which require admission at present but to seek further consultation if things worsen.

If admission is required explain why as clearly and concisely as possible in straightforward language.

Other agencies

If the patient requires admission then a clear, concise, and legible letter to the admitting team is appropriate in all but the imminently life-threatening case (e.g. AAA – abdominal aortic aneurysm). This should include the important details from the history and examination, as well as details of any previous consultations if known.

If the patient is managed at home ensure details are entered in the GP notes or details sent to the patient's GP as appropriate.

Normal labour

If delivery is not imminent transfer to labour ward or contact community midwife. However, the emergency practitioner may be faced with a woman in preterm labour, or with a concealed or unsuspected pregnancy who is about to deliver. The local obstetric unit should be contacted to request an on-call community midwife to attend. A detailed description is found in many texts.[1-3] Management is summarised in Box 9.15. The key action is to provide gentle support.

Syntometrine should be given soon after delivery if it is available as it reduces bleeding and aids separation of the placenta. This should only be given when it is quite certain that this is not a multiple pregnancy.

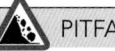

PITFALL

Syntometrine or ergometrine will exacerbate hypertension – use syntocinon instead. None of these drugs should be given if there is a possibility of multiple pregnancy until all babies are delivered

---

BOX 9.15 Summary of the management of normal labour

- If the membranes have broken straw-coloured fluid will be seen; if the fluid is green this may be indicative of fetal compromise, although a small number of green streaks is common
- As the head is delivering ask the woman to pant and only give small pushes
- Put the fingers of one hand against the head to keep it flexed; support the perineum with the other hand
- The head will usually deliver with face looking down towards the mother's buttocks
- Once the head is delivered ask the woman not to push
- Allow the head to turn spontaneously
- Place the hands on either side of the head
- At the next contraction ask the woman to push
- Gently move the head posteriorly to deliver the anterior shoulder
- Once the anterior shoulder is delivered, lift the head anteriorly to deliver the posterior shoulder
- Support the body as it is delivered
- Place the baby on the mother's abdomen
- Dry the baby, discard wet towels and cover with dry towel
- Assess breathing and heart rate; most babies will cry or breathe within 30 seconds and have a rate over 100
- There is no rush to cut the umbilical cord, if all is well then place the cord clamps and cut the cord after it has stopped pulsating
- Palpate the abdomen to ensure that there is only one baby

Multiple births

There is usually a reasonable time delay between delivery of the first baby and the second. The placenta should be left in situ and arrangements made to transfer the mother into an obstetric unit. If the urge to push occurs again delivery should be as detailed elsewhere.

Breech

This is when the feet or bottom are delivered first. You should avoid handling the baby. If necessary any pressure should be placed around the baby's pelvic girdle to ensure that the baby remains with its back uppermost. Ideally the mother should give birth at the edge of the bed so the baby can hang freely to allow gravity to aid delivery. Once the nape of the neck is visible hold the baby's feet and gently sweep them in an upwards arc to a vertical position to aid delivery of the head.

Management of problems

Cord prolapse

If the cord (a rope-like structure) is seen protruding through the vagina the woman should be transported urgently to hospital. If possible she should be placed in an all-fours position with the head down and buttocks up in the air to reduce pressure on the cord and allow oxygen to reach the baby. Put warm saline swabs on the cord (only if readily available – do not delay transport). Warn the receiving unit to prepare for emergency caesarean section.

Shoulder dystocia

After the head delivers, the shoulders should follow within the next two contractions. If they do not deliver *do not* pull on the baby's head, but encourage the mother to push with her hips and knees sharply flexed up towards her shoulders, or alternatively encourage her to turn onto all fours on her hands and knees. Pressure can be put on the anterior shoulder to promote adduction of the shoulders. Stand behind the baby's back and press obliquely downwards above the symphysis pubis.

Post partum haemorrhage

If heavy bleeding occurs IM syntometrine should be given and intravenous access obtained. If the placenta has delivered, the uterus may be aided in its contraction by rubbing the lower abdomen. Make urgent arrangements to transfer into hospital.

Summary

Abdominal pain is a common presentation to the community practitioner. Most presentations can be managed at home with simple advice and support, however some require admission for further assessment.

A structured approach to management will avoid missing the serious signs and symptoms of potentially life-threatening illness. Particular care is required in the very elderly or very young because history taking and examination can be difficult.

References (abdominal pain)

1 Dang C et al 2002 Acute abdominal pain: four classifications can guide assessment and management. Geriatrics 57(3):30–32
2 Simon S, Everitt H, Birtwhistle J, Stevenson B 2002 Oxford handbook of general practice. Oxford University Press, Oxford
3 Greaves I, Dyer P, Porter K 1995 Handbook of immediate care. W B Saunders, London
4 Smail N, Wang P, Cioffi W G, Bland K I, Chaudry I H 1998 Resuscitation after uncontrolled venous hemorrhage: does increased resuscitation volume improve regional perfusion? J Trauma 44:(4)701–708
5 American College Of Emergency Physicians 2000 Clinical policy: critical issues for the initial evaluation and management of patients presenting with a chief complaint of nontraumatic acute abdominal pain. Ann Emerg Med 36(4):406–415
6 Martina B et al 1997 First clinical judgement by primary care physicians distinguishes well between non-organic and organic causes of abdominal or chest pain. J Gen Int Med 12:459

References (pregnancy and its complications)

1 Department of Health 2001 Why Mothers Die 1997–1999 The Fifth Report of the UK Confidential Enquiries into Maternal Deaths. HMSO, London 2001 Available online: http://www.cemach.org.uk/publications.htm (5 Mar 2007)
2 JRCALC 2004 Clinical Practice Guidelines. Available online: http://www.nelh.nhs.uk/emergency (5 Mar 2007)
3 WHO 2000 Managing Complications in Pregnancy and Childbirth. Symptom-based manual. Available online: http://www.who.int/reproductive-health/impac/ (5 Mar 2007)

Carole Gavin and James Gray

Management of neurological emergencies

Introduction

Neurological emergencies are common but require careful assessment to avoid the pitfalls of missing a serious diagnosis, for example headache presents a particular diagnostic challenge, to avoid missing the one subarachnoid haemorrhage amongst the other benign headaches. This chapter discusses the main neurological conditions and outlines assessment and management based upon current best guidance (Box 10.1).

> BOX 10.1 **Conditions covered in this chapter**
>
> ■ The primary survey positive patient
> ■ Fitting – including febrile convulsion
> ■ Headache
> ■ Stroke – including transient ischaemic attacks (TIA)

The primary survey positive patient

The two main problems causing a positive primary survey are the unconscious patient and the fitting patient.

The unconscious patient

It is very difficult to make an accurate neurological assessment of the unconscious patient and these patients will need a full hospital assessment. Call for back up to assist in initial management and transfer.

Ensure the airway is clear and minimise the risk of aspiration by nursing the patient on their side. Give oxygen (15 litres via a non-rebreathing mask) and establish IV access if possible. Transfer to definitive care. Check the blood glucose and assess the Glasgow Coma Score (GCS; Box 10.2). Hypoglycaemia will respond either to 10% glucose IV or IM glucagon administration.

When communicating the GCS to secondary care it can be very usefully broken down into its separate components to give a clear impression of neurological status.

Poisoning and overdose are an important cause of unconsciousness. This is covered more fully in Chapter 14; however it is important that the patient is examined for evidence of IV drug use which might respond to naloxone therapy.

The fitting patient

The fitting patient can provide a significant challenge to the practitioner and attempts should be made to stop the fitting and assess further as required. The National Institute for Health and Clinical Excellence (NICE) has published guidance on fit management[1] (Box 10.3).

Airway management in the fitting patient can be difficult. A nasopharyngeal airway can help provide an airway as oropharyngeal airways may be difficult to use due to jaw spasm. Often parents or carers of patients with frequent fits may already have used rectal diazepam.

Always measure the blood sugar to exclude a hypoglycaemic episode.

If a patient who is a known epileptic has made a full recovery and there is no evidence of injury (to head/shoulder/back), it may be

---

BOX 10.2 **Glasgow Coma Score**

Maximum score = 15, Minimum score = 3
A patient is defined as unconscious with scores ≤8

Eye response
4 – open spontaneously
3 – open to command
2 – open to pain
1 – no eye opening

Verbal response
5 – fluent and orientated
4 – confused speech
3 – inappropriate words
2 – incomprehensible sounds
1 – no verbal response

Motor response
6 – obeys commands
5 – localises to pain
4 – withdraws from pain
3 – flexion to pain
2 – extension to pain
1 – no motor response

BOX 10.3 **NICE guidance on fit management**

If convulsive seizures lasting 5 minutes or longer or three or more seizures in an hour:
- Secure the airway
- Assess respiratory and cardiac function
- Give rectal diazepam in most cases, with buccal midazolam an alternative
- Call emergency services if required by the situation or the response to treatment, and particularly if:
  - seizures develop into status epilepticus
  - there is a high risk of recurrence
  - this is the first episode
  - there may be difficulties monitoring the person's condition

---

possible to leave them at home if they have suitable home support and there is no evidence that the fits are becoming more frequent or associated with another illness. In general all unconscious patients except those who are known to be epileptic, are fully recovered and have a carer at home.

Febrile seizures are any seizure occurring in an infant or young child (6 months to 5 years of age) with a fever, or history of recent fever, and without previous evidence of an afebrile seizure or underlying cause. These occur in between 2–4% of all children at some point and a positive

> **BOX 10.4 Advice to parents following a febrile convulsion**
>
> - A febrile convulsion is due to a fever causing your child to become too hot
> - Febrile convulsions are common, generally harmless and do not indicate epilepsy or cause brain damage
> - They often occur in the first 24 hours of a febrile illness but if they recur the child should be re-evaluated
> - They generally last less than 1 minute but can last longer
> - Simple treatment includes lying your child on its back, removing clothing and sponging with tepid water to cool the child down
> - Do not place anything in the child's mouth
> - They can recur with further febrile illness
> - If the seizure is lasting more than 5 minutes ring 999 for immediate assistance

family history occurs in up to 40%.[2] They can often recur and parental education on treatment can decrease attendance at A&E.

Dealing with these cases can be difficult as parents are often very upset and frightened by the event, requiring a calm and reassuring approach by the healthcare professional. Most children have ceased fitting on arrival and benzodiazepines should be reserved for prolonged seizures – a useful guide is if the child is still fitting on the arrival of assistance. Parents should receive advice regarding febrile seizures after any episode (Box 10.4).

If the episode is a recurrence and the parents are happy and confident in the management of the patient then treatment can be as above at home, with instructions to ring for help if a seizure becomes prolonged.

Headache

The assessment of the patient with headache is difficult even for the most experienced clinician. Headache lends itself very well to assessment via the SOAPC system as by following a careful assessment process an accurate evaluation can be made.[3]

Subjective assessment

The history is often the most important factor in headache assessment with all information assisting in the final evaluation and decision-making (Box 10.5).

- *Headache history*: The patient who has had regular headaches for many years is more likely to have a migrainous or tension type

> BOX 10.5 **Factors to consider in history of a headache**
>
> ■ Headache history
> ■ Frequency and duration of headaches
> ■ Time of onset
> ■ Mode of onset
> ■ Site
> ■ Quality
> ■ Associated symptoms
> ■ Precipitating or aggravating factors
> ■ Relieving factors

headache, while the acute onset of headache in a patient who has never had similar previously may indicate serious pathology such as a subarachnoid haemorrhage. In between is the grey area, which is more difficult to interpret accurately, and must trigger caution.

■ *Frequency and duration*: This is important to distinguish the types of recurrent headache. Migraine often shows a regular pattern of recurrence, while frequent headaches in a short period of time followed by a long, sometimes years, period of remission may indicate cluster headaches. Tension headache has no particular pattern and is often at a background level constantly.

■ *Time of onset*: Migraine often causes the patient to wake whilst cluster headaches often occur at certain times. More serious causes have no specific time pattern.

■ *Mode of onset*: Migraine often has precipitants ranging from an aura (usually visual but may include other focal neurological symptoms), to a feeling of something wrong. Sudden onset or thunderclap headache is suspicious of conditions such as subarachnoid haemorrhage.

■ *Site*: Migraine, cluster headache and trigeminal neuralgia are commonly unilateral whilst tension headache feels like a tight band around the entire head. Subarachnoid haemorrhage can start locally but usually is generalised and may spread to the neck.

■ *Quality*: Headache can be constant, pulsatile or stabbing.

■ *Associated symptoms*: Migraine can commonly give gastrointestinal symptoms, photophobia suggests migraine, meningitis or subarachnoid haemorrhage. Neurological symptoms can occur with migraine but suspicion should be raised about intracranial pathology.

■ *Precipitating and aggravating factors*: Are there any specific triggers the patient can identify? Specific foods, classically chocolate and cheese, can trigger migraine. Aggravation by head movement or coughing/ straining suggests raised intracranial pressure.

■ *Relieving factors*: Patients with a migraine often prefer to lie down in a darkened room whilst patients with cluster headache prefer to move about.

It is important to complete the history with a thorough assessment of the patient's general health and wellbeing including smoking, alcohol and family history.

Objective assessment

Examination of the patient with headache should include a general examination as well as a detailed neurological exam (Box 10.6).

- *General systems examination*: As numerous systemic problems can contribute to headache a full examination is important and may pick up rarer conditions such as endocrine disorders or Marfan's syndrome.
- *Mental state/alertness*: Depressive affect may be apparent, which is a risk for chronic headache conditions. Drowsiness or confusion suggest intracranial pathology or infection.
- *Speech*: Speech disturbance can occur in migraine but a stroke must also be considered.
- *Skull*: In infants the key finding to look for is a bulging fontanelle, which might indicate intracranial pathology. In adults, especially older, palpation of the temporal arteries may reveal evidence of arteritis. Look for evidence of head injury.
- *Neck and other tests*: Neck stiffness usually indicates meningeal irritation from infection or blood. Kernig's and Bradzinski's sign are useful tests for evidence of meningitis.
- *Eyes*: Evidence of glaucoma should be sought as this can present with headache. Fundoscopy should be performed to look for papilloedema or optic atrophy. The cranial nerves controlling eye movements and visual fields can also be tested at this time.
- *ENT*: It is important to ask about loss of smell and examine the ears for any obvious pathology such as otitis media. Many upper respiratory tract infections have a mild headache as part of their presentation and the throat should be examined for signs of tonsillitis.
- *General neurological*: A full generalised neurological examination should be performed in order to finish the patient assessment.

BOX 10.6 **Objective assessment of headache**

- General systems examination
- Mental state/alertness
- Speech
- Skull
- Neck and other tests
- Eyes
- ENT
- General neurological

Analysis

The cause of most headaches will be clear from the history and examination may add little to the differential diagnosis. Box 10.7 gives the common differential diagnosis of headache. In general, all headaches of acute sudden onset will require immediate investigation in secondary care. The subacute causes of headache will require urgent investigation, either immediately if severe enough or in an urgent outpatient assessment.

BOX 10.7 Differential diagnosis of headache

Acute severe
- Subarachnoid haemorrhage
- Meningitis and encephalitis
- Systemic meningism
- Some migraine

Subacute onset
- Expanding intracranial pathology
- Temporal arteritis
- Developing hydrocephalus

Recurrent discrete
- Migraine

Episodic
- Cluster headache
- Trigeminal neuralgia

Chronic headache
- Tension headache
- Migraine
- Post-herpetic neuralgia

Plan and communication

Suspected meningitis, subarachnoid haemorrhage

If the patient has sudden onset of severe headache then they will require immediate secondary care assessment to rule out a sinister cause such as subarachnoid haemorrhage.

If meningitis is suspected then immediate treatment with benzylpenicillin is warranted unless there is a clear history of immediate anaphylactic reaction following administration previously (Fig. 10.1).

In the case of headaches of subacute onset the history and examination should point toward the likely diagnosis. If a space occupying

Fig. 10.1 Treatment of suspected meningitis in the community

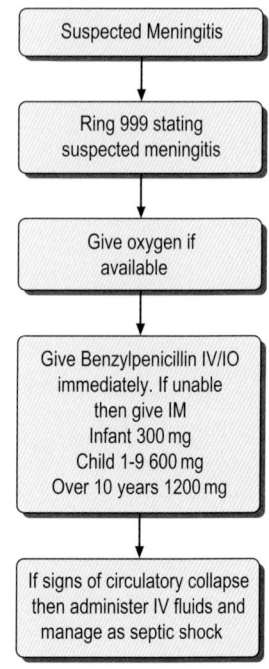

Suspected Meningitis

Ring 999 stating suspected meningitis

Give oxygen if available

Give Benzylpenicillin IV/IO immediately. If unable then give IM
Infant 300 mg
Child 1-9 600 mg
Over 10 years 1200 mg

If signs of circulatory collapse then administer IV fluids and manage as septic shock

lesion is suspected then an urgent neurosurgical consultation is required and consultation with the patient's general practitioner should allow a 2-week wait consult to be arranged.

If migraine is suspected then treatment can be started with a non-steroidal anti-inflammatory medication such as diclofenac along with an anti-emetic such as metoclopramide or, if this has been tried and is unsuccessful, a triptan (e.g. sumatriptan) may be given if the patient is less than 65 years old and has no history of heart disease or hypertension.[4]

If the cause of the headache is not thought to be sinister, reassurance, simple analgesia and referral back to the patient's general practitioner may well be all that is required. In doing so it is important that a communication is made with the GP to alert them to the findings on this occasion so any change at follow-up can be ascertained.

Temporal arteritis

The one other condition to be cautious of is temporal arteritis, which can often present as a headache of unclear cause in patients over 55 years of age. Untreated it can lead to blindness. If suspected on examination then urgent communication of this suspicion with the GP is required to arrange urgent investigation and treatment.

Transient ischaemic attack and stroke

Transient ischaemic attack (TIA) is a clinical syndrome characterised by an acute loss of focal cerebral or ocular function with symptoms lasting less than 24 hours. It is thought to be due to inadequate blood supply to these areas as a result of low flow, thrombosis, or embolism associated with diseases of the blood vessels, heart or blood.

The main concern with TIA is it is associated with very high risk of stroke in the first month following the event and up to one year after. It affects around 35 people per 100 000 per year.

Acute stroke (CVA) is defined as a clinical syndrome, of presumed vascular origin, typified by rapidly developing signs of focal or global disturbance of cerebral function lasting more than 24 hours or leading to death.

Studies put its incidence at 174–216 per 100 000 of the UK population annually and it accounts for 11% of all deaths in England and Wales.[5] Approximately 85% of strokes are due to ischaemia and 15% are due to haemorrhage.

The Intercollegiate Stroke Working Party has set out guidelines for the acute management of stroke and TIA[6] which are used as the basis for this text.

Subjective and objective assessment

History and examination help define if the symptoms are consistent with a focal neurological deficit from brain ischaemia. Symptoms are more usually negative, e.g. loss of function, rather than positive, e.g. tingling or involuntary movements. Non-focal signs and symptoms such as loss of consciousness, dizziness, weakness, confusion and incontinence are rarely due to a TIA.[7]

The most sensitive features associated with diagnosing stroke are facial weakness, arm weakness and speech disturbance, with 80% of strokes demonstrating these three features (the FAST assessment – Box 10.8).[8]

Most areas will have a local protocol for the management of TIA in the acute stages. The difficulty can be distinguishing stroke and TIA in the early stages and unless the patient is clearly recovering hospital assessment is required (Box 10.9). If the patient has recovered then

---

BOX 10.8 **The FAST assessment**

■ Facial weakness
■ Arm weakness
■ Speech Test

BOX 10.9 TIA/stroke symptoms[9]

Anterior circulation
- Unilateral weakness
- Unilateral sensory loss
- Isolated dysarthria
- Dysphasia
- Vision:
  - homonymous hemianopia
  - monocular blindness
  - visual inattention

Posterior circulation
- Isolated homonymous hemianopia
- Diplopia and disconjugate eyes
- Nausea and vomiting
- Inco-ordination and unsteadiness
- Unilateral/bilateral weakness

Non-specific signs
- Dysphagia
- Incontinence
- Loss of consciousness

assessment and investigation should be arranged in a specialist clinic, usually within 7 days. In the meantime it is advised that patients have an anti-platelet commenced, with the evidence favouring aspirin 300 mg immediately followed by 75 mg daily due to the increased risk of stroke in the first few days post TIA. If the patient has recurrent episodes of TIA then the regimen should be changed in line with best practice which would generally recommend the addition of dipyridamole.[10,11] If there is a second TIA within 7 days then the patient requires hospital admission.

There is often little to do in the emergency situation for patients who have had an acute stroke. Those who are unconscious, or primary survey positive, will require appropriate management and immediate transfer to hospital (Box 10.10). Those patients who are not primary survey positive should be assessed using a standard SOAPC approach (see Chapter 2) prior to dispatch to hospital.

BOX 10.10 Patients requiring urgent brain scanning

- Currently taking anticoagulants
- Depressed level of consciousness
- Papilloedema, neck stiffness or fever
- Indications for thrombolysis or early anticoagulation
- Known bleeding tendency
- Unexplained, progressive or fluctuating symptoms
- Severe headache at onset

Important observations should be recorded including blood pressure, pulse, heart rhythm, temperature, blood glucose and, if possible, oxygen saturations. Blood sugar is important as hypoglycaemia or diabetic coma can present with similar features to acute stroke.

Aspirin 300 mg is recommended to be given as soon as possible once a diagnosis of primary haemorrhage has been excluded but, given the difficulty in making this distinction clinically, is not currently recommended in the pre-hospital stages. Thrombolysis in stroke remains a specialist centre procedure and it is unlikely to pass into the pre-hospital arena due to the risks of incorrectly labelling a haemorrhagic stroke as infarction and worsening the haemorrhage.

All patients with a stroke will require hospital assessment for CT scanning and management as appropriate. In some areas there may be facilities for hospital at home management for those patients who are affected by a further stroke with outpatient assessment within 7 days at a hospital clinic. In these few cases local guidelines should be used to guide any treatment such as addition of a second anti-platelet agent.

Summary

Neurological emergencies are seen relatively commonly by the community practitioner, headache providing the most difficult diagnostic challenge and thus causing the greatest uncertainty.

This chapter aims to guide management and is based on the main current guidance but it is clear that with the exception of some headaches and TIA most patients will require secondary care assessment.

All of these conditions however are extremely frightening to both patient and relatives/carer and reassurance and support remains a crucial role for the primary care professional, which can improve the overall management.

References

1 National Institute for Health and Clinical Excellence 2004 The epilepsies: diagnosis and management of the epilepsies in adults in primary and secondary care. NICE, London
2 Warden C R et al 2003 Evaluation and management of febrile seizures in the out-of-hospital and emergency department settings. Ann Emerg Med 41:215–222
3 Lance J W, Goadsby P J 1999 Mechanism and management of headache. Butterworth-Heinemann, Oxford
4 Goadsby P J et al 2002 Migraine – current understanding and treatment. N Engl J Med 346:257–268
5 Mant J et al 2004 Health care needs assessment: the epidemiologically based needs assessment reviews, 2nd edn. Radcliffe Medical Press, Oxford

6 Intercollegiate Stroke Working Party 2004 National clinical guidelines for stroke, 2nd edn. Royal College of Physicians, London

7 Shah K, Edlow J 2004 Transient ischaemic attack: review for the emergency physician. Ann Emerg Med 43:592–603

8 Joint Royal Colleges Ambulance Liason Committee & Todd I (ed) 2004 Clinical practice guidelines for use in UK ambulance services. JRCALC, London. Available online:http://www.nelh.nhs.uk/emergency (5 Mar 2007)

9 Bath P M W, Lees K R 2000 ABC of arterial and venous disease – acute stroke. BMJ 320:920–923

10 Tran H, Anand S 2004 Oral antiplatelet therapy in cerebrovascular disease, coronary artery disease, and peripheral arterial disease. JAMA 292:1867–1874

11 Antithrombotic Trialists' Collaboration 2002 Collaborative meta-analysis of randomised trials of antiplatelet therapy for prevention of death, myocardial infarction, and stroke in high risk patients. BMJ 324:71–86

Sarah Carter and Colville Laird

ENT problems

Introduction

The vast majority of ENT (ear, nose and throat) problems that present in the pre-hospital setting are minor in nature. However, occasionally innocuous symptoms can develop into life-threatening conditions which require immediate assessment and treatment. The objectives of this chapter are outlined in Box 11.1.

Primary survey

The primary survey (Box 11.2) is a rapid assessment tool which uses the ABC principles to look for an immediately life-threatening condition.

BOX 11.1 Chapter objectives

- To undertake a primary survey of the patient and treat any immediately life-threatening problems
- To identify any patients who have a normal primary survey but have an obvious need for hospital admission
- To undertake a secondary survey (full assessment) including history and examination targeted to the presenting symptom
- To consider a list of differential diagnoses
- Discuss treatment based on the likely diagnosis(es) and whether home management or hospital admission is appropriate
- Consider need for follow-up

BOX 11.2 Primary survey

If any observations below are present treat immediately and transfer to hospital:
- Airway obstruction
- Respiratory rate <10 or >29
- O_2 sats <93%
- Pulse <50 or >120
- Systolic BP <90
- GCS <12

ENT conditions can be immediately life-threatening by causing an A, B or C problem:

- **A** Airway obstruction/compromise – inhaled foreign body, epiglottitis, quinsy, anaphylaxis/angio-oedema, croup, facial fractures
- **B** Breathing difficulty – croup, inhaled foreign body
- **C** Circulatory compromise – haemorrhage, e.g. epistaxis, from facial fracture, secondary haemorrhage following ENT surgery, e.g. post-tonsillectomy.

Patients with a normal primary survey but with obvious need for hospital admission

Patients with all of the above conditions can show a spectrum of severity of symptoms and signs, which can deteriorate. It is essential to remember that in the early stages of these conditions, patients may not have significant abnormal physical signs. The recognition of developing airway obstruction is critical and management of the condition may require the use of airway adjuncts to maintain adequate oxygenation. If there is complete airway obstruction and airway adjuncts have failed, prompt insertion of a surgical airway may be required as a last resort. It is important to monitor patients with respiratory distress for deterioration and exhaustion. In the case of haemorrhage the body will initially compensate. Therefore cases leading to hypovolaemia should be treated by arresting the haemorrhage and administering fluid to maintain a radial pulse.

The history and a brief examination may lead you to suspect that one of the above conditions is the likely diagnosis and problems with the airway, breathing or circulation may develop. All suspected cases of:

- foreign body inhalation
- epiglottitis
- anaphylaxis
- posterior nasal haemorrhage
- unstable facial fractures
- secondary haemorrhage post surgery

should be admitted to hospital for further investigation and management. However, not all cases of croup or epistaxis will require hospital admission. Management of the individual conditions is discussed below or in other chapters of this book.

Secondary survey

Patients still remaining after the primary survey require a thorough assessment to determine optimal treatment and discharge (see Chapter 2).

- *History and examination*. Should be targeted to the presenting symptom and associated systems. Examination of the respiratory and cardiovascular systems is always necessary. This should be supplemented with abdominal assessment when glandular fever is suspected, looking for hepatosplenomegaly, and examination of the central nervous system if vertigo or facial weakness is the presenting symptom.
- *Vital signs*. Unless you are transporting the patient immediately, then always measure a full set of vital signs.
- *Investigations*. Other than a full history and examination there are no investigations available in the pre-hospital setting able to confirm or refute any of the differential diagnoses.

Differential diagnosis

Table 11.1 shows details of the differential diagnoses classified by presenting symptom.

TABLE 11.1 Differential diagnoses classified by presenting symptom

Presenting symptom	ENT diagnoses	Other differential diagnoses
Nose bleed	Anterior bleed Posterior bleed Traumatic Post surgery	Underlying bleeding disorder
Sore throat	Tonsillitis Pharyngitis Glandular fever Candida Quinsy Stevens–Johnson syndrome Ramsey–Hunt syndrome	Angina Gastro-oesophageal reflux Tobacco usage Occupational irritants
Sore ears	Otitis externa Viral otitis media Bacterial otitis media Perforated tympanic membrane Eustachian tube dysfunction Mastoiditis Ramsey–Hunt syndrome	Temporomandibular joint dysfunction Upper GI and airway neoplasms Dental Cervical spondylosis
Foreign body	Ears Nose Airway	
Difficult/noisy breathing	Foreign body Epiglottitis Croup Anaphylaxis Bacterial tracheitis Smoke inhalation	Asthma COPD
Vertigo	Vestibular neuronitis Meniere's Benign paroxysmal positional vertigo	Cerebellar CVA Other central causes
Facial/tooth pain	Sinusitis Dental abscess	Shingles Trigeminal neuralgia
Facial weakness	Bells palsy Ramsey–Hunt syndrome	CVA
Sudden hearing loss	Wax impaction Perforated TM	CVA
Trauma	Facial fractures Perforated TM	

Presenting symptoms, history, examination and treatment

Nose bleed

The following points in the history are important for the management of a patient with a nose bleed:

- age of patient
- number of bleeding episodes
- sensation of blood in the throat
- amount of blood/duration of bleeding
- previous history of epistaxis, trauma, nasal surgery
- family history of bleeding disorder
- anticoagulant, NSAID, aspirin, cocaine use
- other significant medical conditions, e.g. IHD, COPD, hypertension, coagulopathy.

When examining the patient try to locate the side of the bleeding, look at the linearity of the nose (if asymmetrical, is this due to recent trauma?); check the appearance of the septum and Little's area. The latter is the area of the septum seen through the nostrils when the nasal tip is tilted upwards (Fig. 11.1). Blood vessels in Little's area are prone to bleeding. Check the throat for blood running down the nasopharynx. Ensure you get a set of vital signs and examine the cardiovascular system looking for any indication of shock.

The treatment of epistaxis is dependent on the site of the bleeding and the experience of the healthcare professional.

If bleeding has stopped by the time of presentation or ceases with the simple first aid measures (TIP) and the vital signs are normal no further treatment is necessary. If it is a recurrent bleed antibiotic nasal cream should be prescribed. Recurrent nose bleeds in children tend to be caused by digital trauma to Little's area. In adults remember to check blood pressure. If elevated, ask them to attend the GP for further management.

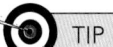

TIP

The majority of nose bleeds will respond to simple first aid measures of compression and cooling. It is important to note that effective compression occludes both nostrils without release, for 20 minutes. Cooling with a cold compress over the forehead and bridge of the nose can also be effective by causing vasoconstriction of the nasal vessels

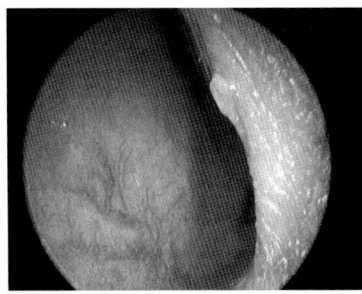

Fig. 11.1 Little's area of the nasal septum (reproduced with permission of Mr Kim Ah-See, ENT Consultant, Aberdeen).

If the bleeding fails to respond to simple first aid measures packing should be applied to the nasal cavity from which the bleed is suspected to have originated. The simplest pack and the easiest to insert is the nasal tampon (Fig. 11.2). However, the nose can be packed with ribbon gauze if available and the healthcare professional is competent at the procedure. Nasal tampons are supplied small and flat but expand and take on the contours of the cavity when they are hydrated with either blood or saline. The leading edge of the nasal tampon should be lubricated prior to insertion. It should then be inserted in a horizontal plane into the nasal cavity. If the nasal tampon does not expand with the blood in the nose, saline should be dripped onto the external end of the nasal tampon until it expands and causes compression. The thread of the tampon should be secured with tape and a nasal sling may be applied to soak up any excess blood.

If anterior packing fails to stop the bleeding after 15 minutes a posterior bleed should be suspected (approx. 5% of bleeds). These require packing using a long nasal tampon, an epistaxis balloon or a Foley catheter with an anterior pack depending on what is available (Fig. 11.3). Long (posterior) nasal tampons are inserted in the same way as an anterior tampon. Some epistaxis balloons have an anterior and posterior balloon. The balloon is lubricated with saline and inserted, again in a horizontal plane. The posterior balloon is inflated to the recommended volume, gentle traction is applied to position the balloon in the posterior nasal space and then the anterior balloon is inflated to the recommended volume. Foley catheters and single balloon epistaxis catheters are inserted in the same way but do not have an anterior balloon and therefore an anterior pack is necessary. The Foley catheter must be secured with care taken to prevent pressure necrosis of the nasal tissues. *All patients with a posterior bleed require admission* (Box 11.3). If a large volume of blood has been lost, oxygen, venous access and fluid resuscitation may be necessary.

TIP

For healthcare professionals with additional skills. If the bleeding point can be visualised cautery of the vessel can be attempted with either silver nitrate or electrocautery if available. Cautery should be applied to a specific vessel and not used in a blanket fashion to the nasal mucosa. If the bleeding source is not visible, or cautery fails, then the nose should be packed with an anterior pack

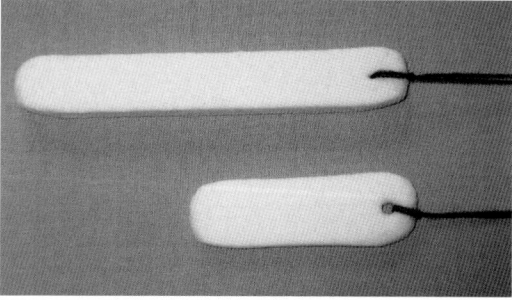

Fig. 11.2   Nasal tampon (reproduced with permission of BASICS Scotland).

Fig. 11.3 Posterior and anterior nasal tampons, deflated and inflated double balloon epistaxis catheters and single posterior space epistaxis balloon catheter (reproduced with permission of BASICS Scotland).

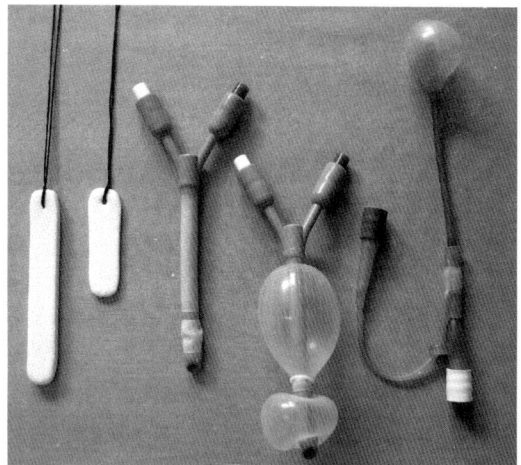

BOX 11.3 Patients with a nose bleed – who needs to go to hospital?

- All patients with a posterior pack must be admitted to hospital. They require analgesia and close monitoring particularly of vital signs and O$_2$ saturations
- All patients with a personal history of bleeding disorder must be admitted to hospital
- Patients with a history of recent nasal surgery should be discussed with the appropriate surgical team
- Patients taking anticoagulants may be treated in the community if a recent INR is known and over-anticoagulation is not suspected
- Patients with an anterior pack and significant other medical illness such as angina or COPD should be considered for admission for close monitoring depending on severity of co-morbid conditions. By packing the patient's nose we cause respiratory compromise that may lead to exacerbations of pre-existing illnesses
- Epistaxis precipitated by trauma and where a facial or nasal fracture cannot be excluded should be referred to hospital

Sore throat

Several features need to be elicited when dealing with patients with sore throats:

- duration?
- previous episodes or recent surgery?
- response to previous treatments?

- one side or both?
- associated features or other symptoms (associated symptoms may lead to a particular diagnosis)?
- ability to swallow food, liquid, saliva?
- halitosis?
- drugs which may cause agranulocytosis, candidal overgrowth or Stevens–Johnson syndrome?
- occupational exposure to physical irritants?

When examining the throat look at the appearance of the tonsils and surrounding tissue. If swelling is present, is it bilateral or unilateral? Is there pus or exudate present on the tonsils (tonsillitis or glandular fever)? If the patient has had recent tonsillar surgery does the tonsillar bed look sloughy, infected or bleeding? Is there peritonsilar redness or swelling (peritonsilar cellulitis)? Look at the appearance of the pharynx – does it look red (pharyngitis), are there any white spots (candida) or ulcerated areas? Can the patient swallow or are they drooling saliva? Is trismus (spasm of the pterygoid muscles preventing opening of the mouth) present (quinsy)? Does the patient have features of systemic toxicity or lymph nodes?

Pharyngitis/tonsillitis/glandular fever/candida

Most sore throats (90–95%) are viral in nature and require only symptomatic treatment with fluids and an antipyretic analgesic. Mild cases of *bacterial tonsillitis*, commonly from streptococci, will also respond to this conservative treatment. However, if the patient has significant fever, nausea and vomiting and no signs of a viral URTI (upper respiratory tract infection) the use of antibiotics can be argued. The choice of antibiotic should be penicillin V or erythromycin initially for 10 days. Shorter treatment durations have been associated with recurrent and early relapse of the infection.

There is no test available to differentiate *glandular fever* from tonsillitis at initial emergency presentation. Therefore the initial treatment is the same as for tonsillitis. Amoxicillin based antibiotics should be avoided if glandular fever is suspected as it can cause a generalised macular rash. If the patient is unable to swallow fluids or their own saliva hospital admission for assessment and intravenous antibiotics will be necessary.

Candidal sore throats can be suspected on history and confirmed on examination by the presence of white plaques adherent to the mucosa of the palate and gums (Fig. 11.4). Treatment is with a topical antifungal such as nystatin. If the patient is immunocompromised then systemic antifungals may be necessary.

Peritonsillar cellulitis and quinsy

Both of these conditions are complications of bacterial tonsillitis and should be suspected in someone whose sore throat gets substantially

Fig. 11.4 Candidal infection of throat (reproduced with permission of the BMJ Publishing Group from Emerg Med J 2005 22:128–139).

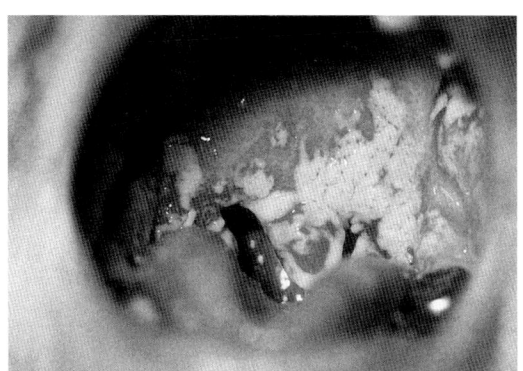

worse and who becomes more unwell than is usual with an uncomplicated tonsillitis. Peritonsillar cellulitis is the presuppurative stage of quinsy – a localised collection of pus above the tonsil. A patient with either condition will complain of a severe unilateral sore throat and difficulty swallowing. The patient may also complain of ipsilateral (on the same side) ear pain and pain on movement of the neck. Examination of the throat will reveal a very swollen, red area above and to the side of the inflamed tonsil. The uvula (the tissue that hangs down from the roof of the mouth at the back of the palate) may be pushed to one side. Enlarged cervical lymph nodes are the cause of the neck pain. If peritonsillar cellulitis is the diagnosis there will be relatively little trismus. If trismus is a feature, quinsy should be suspected. There may be a change to the quality of the voice. Treatment may require drainage, intravenous antibiotics and fluids. Suspected cases need to be referred to hospital for assessment and treatment (Box 11.4).

Stevens–Johnson syndrome

This is a rare multisystem illness with widespread vesiculobullous lesions and erosions of the mucous membranes associated with erythema

---

BOX 11.4 Patients with a sore throat – who needs to go to hospital?

■ Patients with severe tonsillitis with systemic upset and inability to swallow should be admitted for IV antibiotics and fluid. Pain on swallowing, on its own, is not an indication for hospital admission
■ Patients with quinsy should be admitted to hospital for incision and drainage
■ Patients with suspected Stevens–Johnson syndrome should be admitted to hospital

multiforme of the skin (Fig. 11.5). The highest incidence is in the 20–40-year age group; it is twice as common in males and is more common in spring and autumn. Infection (especially *Mycoplasma* and herpes simplex), drugs (especially antibiotics and anticonvulsants) and malignancies are common precipitating factors; 50% of cases have no identifiable aetiology. Suspected cases should be referred to hospital for assessment as many will require ITU or HDU care.

Ramsey–Hunt syndrome
See below.

Non-ENT causes of sore throat
- *Angina* can present with pain in the throat or jaw related to physical exertion. Consider this in middle aged and older patients, with or without a previous history of ischaemic heart disease, with a normal throat examination and no other ENT symptoms. Patients with suspected angina should have an ECG and be given sublingual nitrate (see Chapter 3).
- *Gastro-oesophageal reflux disease* can present with a sore throat and persistent cough. Examination often reveals pharyngitis. Consider this in older, overweight individuals with a persistent sore throat with or without a history of dyspepsia.
- *Tobacco usage* – heavy smokers may develop a chronic pharyngitis with pain.
- *Occupational irritants* – fumes from some chemicals can cause a chronic pharyngitis.

Figure 11.6 shows the sore throat treatment algorithm.

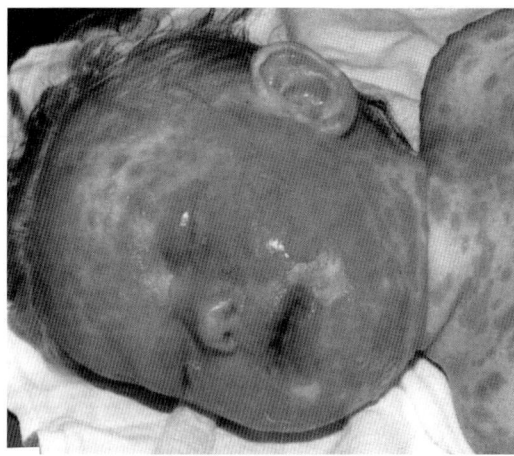

Fig. 11.5 Stevens–Johnson syndrome (reproduced with permission of the BMJ Publishing Group from Emerg Med J 2005 22:128–139).

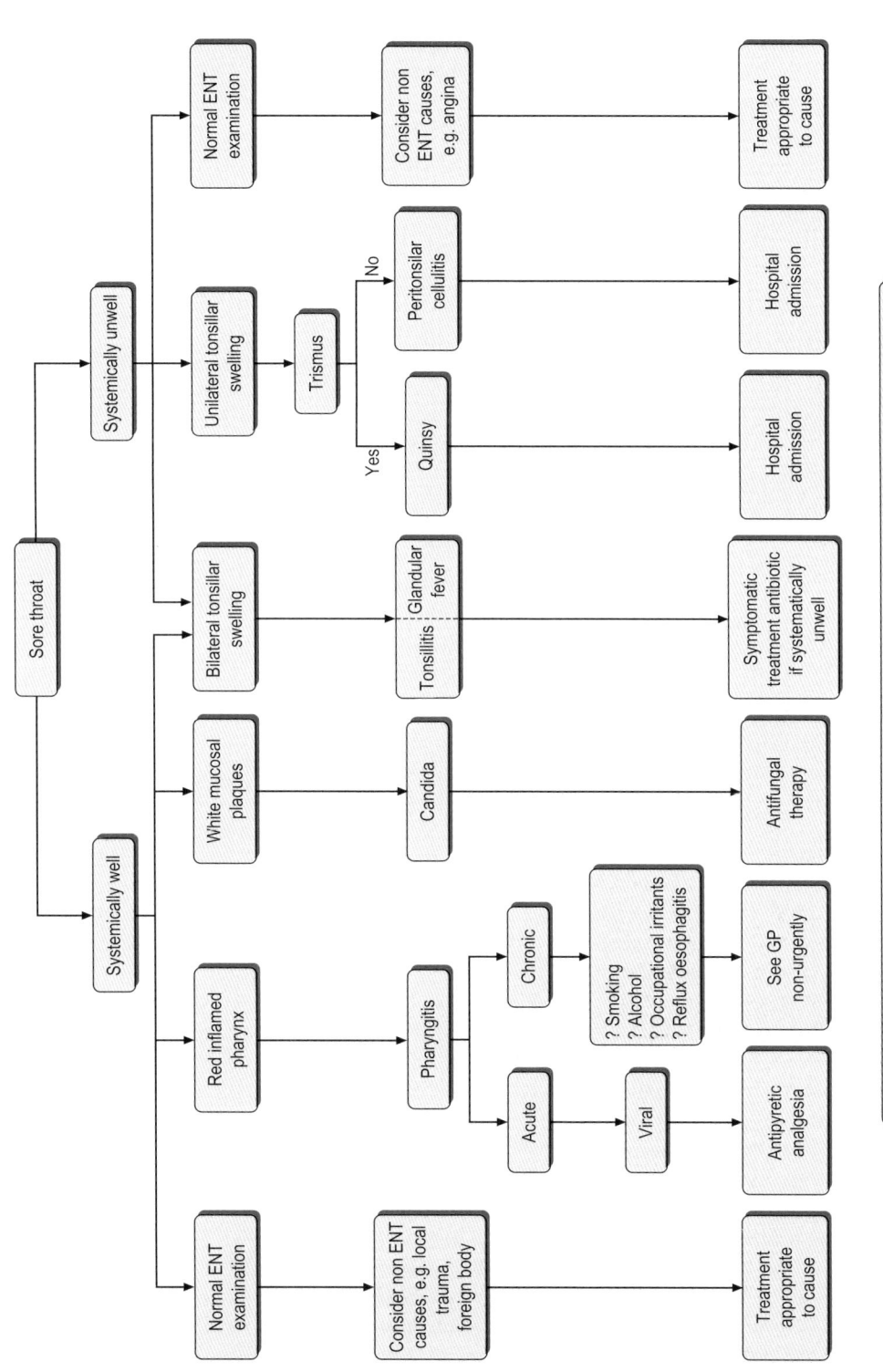

Fig. 11.6 Sore throat treatment algorithm.

Sore ears/discharging ears

Painful ears are a common complaint, particularly in young children. The pain may originate from the ear itself or be referred from another site. There are some important features to establish about the pain to help make the diagnosis:

- is there a discharge?
- associated symptoms, e.g. coryza, symptoms of systemic toxicity?
- one ear or both?
- previous episodes, previous surgery or recent ear syringing?
- do you use cotton buds?
- recent swimming, diving or flying?
- is there any associated hearing loss?

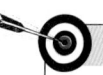

> **TIP**
>
> Always examine the non-painful ear first

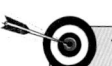

> **TIP**
>
> Try http://www.rcsullivan.com for many video otoscopy images

When examining the ear look for the presence of scars; for deformity of the pinna; at the appearance of external auditory canals; at the appearance of tympanic membranes. Feel for lymph nodes. Does tugging on the pinna or pressure on the tragus cause discomfort (otitis externa/furunculosis) – look behind the pinna at the skin over the mastoid process for swelling or redness; feel for tenderness (mastoiditis).

Otitis externa/furunculosis

Otitis externa is an inflammation (usually infective) of the external auditory canal, which can spread to the pinna, periauricular soft tissues, or even the temporal bone. It is common in patients with eczematous ear canal skin and in those who produce trauma with cotton buds. Streptococci, staphylococci, pseudomonas and fungi are the usual infecting organisms. Pressure on the tragus or gentle tugging on the pinna (Fig. 11.7) will cause discomfort. In the early stages the canal is tender and red and there may be a slight watery discharge. As the condition progresses there may be oedema of the canal and accumulation of debris. Treatment is with topical antibiotic and steroid combination drops and simple analgesia. Any associated cellulitis should be treated with systemic antibiotics.

Furunculosis is an infection of a hair follicle. When this occurs in the outer ear canal it causes severe throbbing pain. Examination of the ear canal may reveal a red lump with or without pus. The abscess may rupture itself or may in severe cases require incision and drainage. Simple analgesia is the only initial treatment necessary with advice to see the GP if not improving within 48 hours.

Otitis media

Acute otitis media (AOM) is usually a short-term inflammation of the middle ear and is principally characterised by earache, irritability and ear tugging in children. Loss of hearing may also occur due to effusion in the middle ear. It is often preceded by upper respiratory symptoms, including

Fig. 11.7 Tugging on the pinna in an upward and backward direction to try and elicit discomfort caused by external auditory canal problems (reproduced with permission of BASICS Scotland).

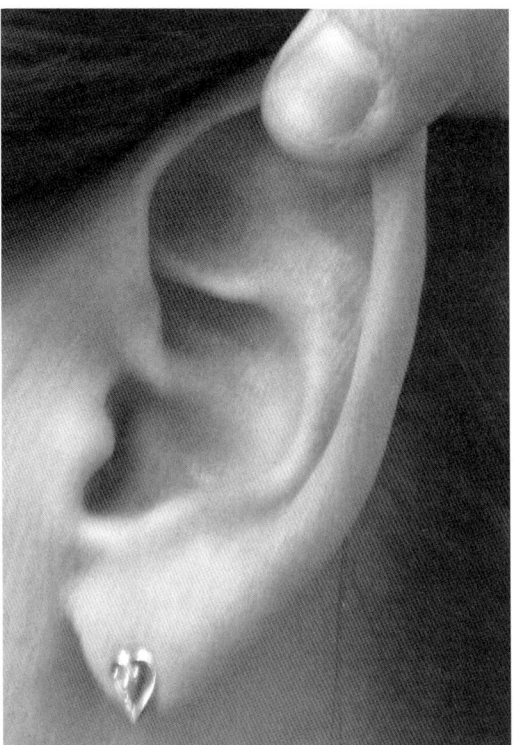

cough and rhinorrhoea. Systemic symptoms can also be present depending on the severity of the illness. Otoscopic appearances typical of AOM include bulging tympanic membrane with loss of landmarks, changes in membrane colour (typically red or yellow) and perforated tympanic membrane with discharge of pus.

The cause of acute otitis media may be viral or bacterial in origin. Viruses are present in about 40–75% of infections and often precede or co-exist with bacterial infections. The main bacteria responsible are *Streptococcus pneumoniae* (40%), *Haemophilus influenzae* (25%) and *Moraxella cattarhalis* (10%). Effusion is a common complication of AOM but severe complications including mastoiditis are exceedingly rare. Mastoiditis has been found to occur in less than 1 in 1000 children with untreated AOM.

AOM is usually a self-limiting condition. About 80% of AOM will resolve within 3 days without antibiotic treatment. Although there is no definitive consensus on the optimum treatment of AOM in children, the available evidence suggests that antibiotic treatment should not be offered routinely. The mainstay of treatment is analgesia. Both paracetamol and ibuprofen are adequate analgesics. Parents should be reassured and involved in discussions of the pros and cons of antibiotic treatment. A 'wait and see' approach may be a good compromise for some people. A prescription for antibiotics can be issued on the day of consultation but not be redeemed unless the condition has not resolved after 72 hours. This has been found to be effective and feasible in two studies.[1,2] Although antibiotics should not be routinely prescribed, the following indications may support their selective use:

- child under 2 years
- bilateral AOM
- systemic symptoms including high temperature and vomiting
- local signs (such as tympanic perforation and discharge of pus) that suggest the infection is severe.

The recommended antibiotics for uncomplicated AOM are shown in Table 11.2.

There is currently no consensus on the optimal length of treatment with antibiotics for acute otitis media; however the available evidence (Box 11.5) suggests that a 5-day course of antibiotics is usually adequate with the exception of azithromycin where 3 days use is sufficient because of its unique pharmacokinetics. The treatment of AOM with antihistamines and decongestants is not recommended.

Perforated tympanic membrane

Tympanic perforations may be secondary to acute otitis media or trauma. Examination of the ear shows loss of the cone of light as the light usually

TABLE 11.2 Recommended antibiotics for uncomplicated AOM		
Antibiotic treatment	AOM first line	AOM second line (treatment failure)
No penicillin allergy	Amoxicillin	Co-amoxiclav
Penicillin allergy	Azithromycin Erythromycin Clarithromycin	Azithromycin if erythromycin used first-line OR seek specialist advice from local microbiologist

---

BOX 11.5 **Evidence for the treatment of otitis media**

- The 2004 SIGN guideline on otitis media[3] found that 17 children need to be given antibiotics for one child to benefit from resolution of symptoms
- A Cochrane review[4] gave the NNT as approximately 15
- Another systematic review[5] including more studies of younger children suggests the NNT is 8
- The clinical impact of antibiotic treatment in children under 2 years of age may be greater than in older children[6] but the frequency of adverse effects seen with antibiotics used to treat AOM may be as high as the NNT required to produce a clinical benefit[7,8]

reflects off the tympanic membrane. Perforations may be partial or total. Partial perforations are easier to recognise than total perforations. Those associated with acute otitis media and profuse discharge of pus should be treated with antibiotics. Traumatic perforations do not require initial treatment. All patients with perforations should be told not to put anything in the ear and not to submerge the ear under water. Not all perforations will heal, therefore follow-up by the GP 10–14 days later is required – or sooner if new symptoms develop.

Mastoiditis

This is a complication of acute otitis media. Presentation is usually of severe pain over the mastoid process and the patient being systemically unwell. Early signs include oedema and redness over the mastoid and oedema of the posterior ear canal wall which is seen as a bulging or sagging of the posterior wall as you look into the external auditory meatus. In severe cases the pinna can be pushed forward. This condition must be referred to hospital for treatment.

Ramsey–Hunt syndrome

Herpes zoster infection of the motor ganglia of the 7th cranial nerve (facial nerve) produces a facial nerve palsy associated with the typical shingles rash in the ear and often on the soft palate and loss of taste on the anterior two-thirds of the tongue. Patients with this condition must be discussed with a senior ENT surgeon or referred back to their own GP if symptoms are not severe.

Non-ENT causes of ear pain

If there is nothing to find on physical examination of the ear the pain may be referred. There are no causes which need out-of-hours treatment but the patient requires simple analgesia and should be told to see their own GP for further assessment.

Figure 11.8 shows the sore ear treatment algorithm.

Foreign body

Foreign bodies in the nose and ear are common in children. A foreign body in the nose, unless impacted, may be inhaled and cause airway compromise. The best way of removal from the nose is to encourage the patient to blow it out themselves, although this can be very difficult in children. An alternative is to cause pressure behind the object to dislodge it. This can be done either by the parent blowing into the child's mouth whilst occluding the unaffected nostril or by using a bag valve mask to produce the pressure. The swift puff of air forces the foreign body down the nostril. If this does not work and there is a risk of inhalation further assistance should be sought. Foreign bodies in ears are not such a potential problem and routine attendance to GP or A&E is sufficient advice.

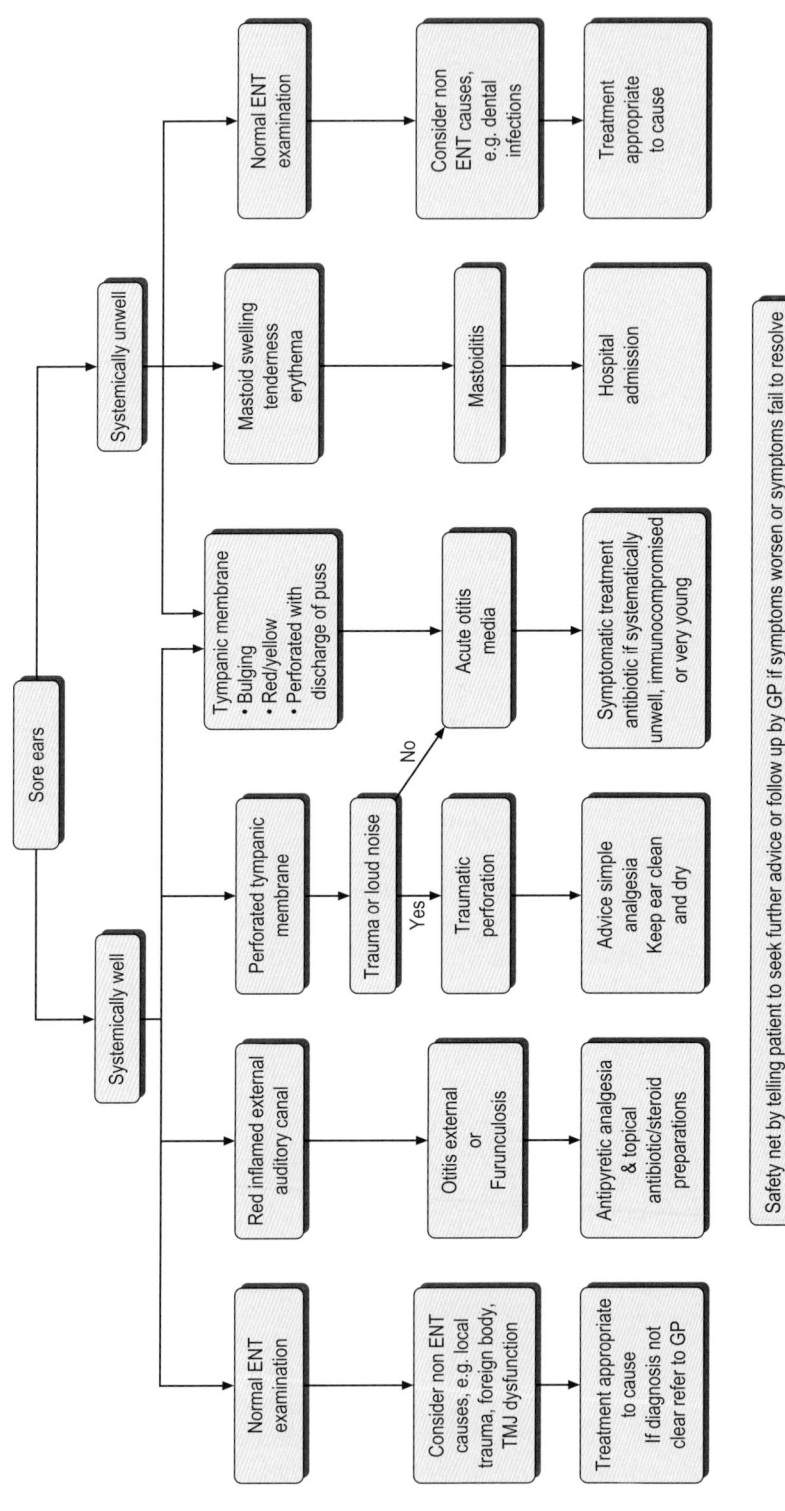

Fig. 11.8 Sore ear treatment algorithm.

Difficult/noisy breathing

See Table 11.3

Epiglottitis

This is a life-threatening condition caused by *Haemophilus influenzae* infection of the epiglottis. It is now much less common since the advent of Hib vaccination but can occur in those who have not been immunised. Though usually seen in 3–7-year-olds it can occur in adults. The onset of symptoms is rapid with high fever and sore throat being the earliest features. The patient can then develop stridor (a harsh, high-pitched, musical sound produced by turbulent airflow through a partially obstructed airway) and the voice may be muffled or absent. Tachycardia, tachypnoea, swallowing difficulties and drooling may then ensue. The patient will appear toxic, apprehensive and pale. Often they sit upright, leaning forward with neck extended, mouth open and jaw thrust forward – in an attempt to maximise the diameter of the airway. There is usually no cough. Cyanosis, shock, loss of consciousness and complete airway obstruction will ensue unless intervention by a senior ENT surgeon is instigated immediately. **Do not attempt to examine the throat.** Refer immediately to a hospital with ENT facilities and warn of suspected diagnosis. Give oxygen but do not

TABLE 11.3 Causes and symptoms of difficult and/or noisy breathing						
	Epiglottitis	Croup	Bacterial tracheitis	Foreign body inhalation	Smoke inhalation	Asthma
Age group	3–7 years commonest	6 months to 3 years	Any	Any	Any	Any
Ill/systemic toxicity	Yes	No	Yes	No	No	No
Pyrexia	Yes	Yes/No	Yes	No	No	No
Sudden onset	Yes	No	No	Yes	History of contact	Yes/No
Cough	Unlikely	Yes	Yes	Yes/No	Yes/No	Yes/No
Stridor	Yes	Yes	Yes	Yes/No	Yes/No	No
Sore throat	Yes	Yes/No	Yes/No	No	No	No
Altered voice	Yes	No	Yes	No	Yes/No	No
Drooling	Yes	No	No	Yes/No	No	No

cause distress and allow the patient to maintain their upright posture. Be prepared to manage the airway en route if necessary. Continue to reassess ABCs during transfer.

Croup

Laryngotracheobronchitis is usually a viral infection. It may be mild or severe and the child can quickly develop respiratory distress. Occurring mainly between the ages of 6 months and 3 years you should suspect if there is pyrexia, a painful barking cough and stridor. All children under the age of 1 year should be admitted to hospital. If there are features of severe respiratory distress (Box 11.6) the child should be admitted to hospital irrespective of age.

Steroid treatment should be initiated if not admitting the child. A single dose of soluble prednisolone 20 mg or alternative can be given. The child should be reassessed 2–4 h later to ensure the stridor is not worsening. If there is severe airway obstruction nebulised epinephrine (5 ml of 1:10000 or 1 ml of 1:1000 diluted to 5 ml with saline) can be given and rapid transport arranged. Severe respiratory distress can come on quickly and the healthcare professional should be prepared to intubate and ventilate in the case of respiratory arrest.

BOX 11.6 **Features of severe respiratory distress**

- Cyanosis
- Agitation
- Extreme dyspnoea
- SpO_2 <93% in air
- Marked use of accessory muscles with marked intercostal and subcostal recession and fatigue

---

Bacterial tracheitis

Stridor, hoarse voice and cough associated with a high fever and a toxic ill-looking child without swallowing difficulties suggests bacterial tracheitis. These children should be admitted to hospital.

Smoke inhalation

Smoke inhalation may be mild, moderate or severe. If associated with other injuries the patient should be sent to hospital for a full assessment. The signs and symptoms of injury may not be immediately apparent but suspect an airway burn and the potential for the patient to develop airway obstruction if the patient has singed eyebrows and singed nasal hair. The important signs to look for are increased respiratory rate, hoarseness, stridor and carbonaceous sputum. If any of these are present give 100% O_2 and arrange transfer to hospital for further assessment.

Non-ENT causes of difficult/noisy breathing

Asthma and COPD are covered in Chapter 4.

Vertigo[9]

Vertigo, an illusion of movement, is the cardinal symptom of vestibular dysfunction. Vertigo is typically rotational, but it can be an illusion of tilting to one side or swaying. It is common for acute vertigo to cause a feeling of imbalance during standing or walking. Patients want to lie still and avoid movement. Acute vertigo is accompanied by nausea, vomiting, and autonomic distress of varying degrees of severity. The difficulty is separating the peripheral (otogenic) causes from a central cause (Table 11.4). Peripheral conditions causing vertigo can include external auditory canal obstruction, middle ear infection or trauma, Meniere's disease and vestibular neuronitis. Central problems presenting with vertigo are usually more serious than the peripheral ones and can include cerebellar infarct or haemorrhage, intracranial space-occupying lesions and demyelinating disease.

Some additional questions in the history may help:

■ duration of the vertigo and rate of onset?
■ associated hearing loss and/or tinnitus?
■ is the vertigo precipitated by rapid head movement?
■ any previous ear problems, trauma or surgery?

A detailed examination of the ear and central nervous system (particularly looking for cerebellar signs) is required (Box 11.7). The type of nystagmus, presence of cerebellar or other neurological symptoms or signs, presence of risk factors for stroke and ability of the patient to walk may help to reach a diagnosis (Fig. 11.10).

TABLE 11.4 Differentiating between peripheral and central vestibular disorder	
Peripheral vestibular disorder	**Central vestibular disorder**
Nystagmus – horizontal with a tortional component – increase in intensity when gaze to side of fast phase – nystagmus can be controlled by fixation Normal CNS examination Unsteady gait lean or fall to side opposite the fast phase of nystagmus	Nystagmus – gaze evoked – horizontal, vertical or tortional – nystagmus can not be controlled by fixation May be: – cranial nerve signs – cerebellar signs – motor weakness – other CNS disturbance May be unable to walk without falling

BOX 11.7 Cerebellar examination

Nystagmus

Assess for nystagmus, a rhythmical beating/flickering of the eye on movement of the eye. Nystagmus at extremes of gaze is not pathological. Peripheral vestibular nystagmus continues in the same direction when the direction of gaze changes. The direction is typically horizontal, with a tortional (rotational) component, it increases in intensity when the gaze is in the direction of the fast phase, and decreases in intensity when the gaze is away from the fast phase (Alexander's law). The intensity and the velocity of its slow phase are attenuated by visual fixation and increased by removing fixation. Acute central disorders, such as infarction or haemorrhage of the brain stem or the cerebellum, may cause spontaneous nystagmus that changes its direction with a change in the direction of gaze (gaze-evoked nystagmus). However, in patients with cerebellar stroke, nystagmus may be present only when the patient is gazing in one direction, thereby appearing similar to a peripheral vestibular nystagmus. Purely vertical nystagmus (nystagmus on looking up and down) and purely torsional nystagmus are almost always due to a central disorder, whereas horizontal and torsional components may occur simultaneously in patients with either peripheral or central disorders. Visual fixation may have little effect on the intensity of central vestibular nystagmus.

Gait ataxia

When trying to walk the patient is unsteady, often repeatedly stumbling to the same side. To detect a more subtle disturbance of cerebellar function ask the patient to heel–toe walk. Remember however that the elderly patient may already have a gait disturbance or loss of confidence.

Co-ordination tests

Always remember to assess one side against the other and not in relation to yourself. For ease of explanation show the patient what you want them to do.

Finger–nose test. Ask the patient to touch their nose with a single finger then to touch your finger held about 0.5 m in front of them. Repeat this moving your finger to a different position. Ask the patient to complete the task as quickly as they can. A patient with a cerebellar problem will demonstrate an intention tremor and past pointing (missing the target) (Fig. 11.9).

Hand tapping test. Ask the patient to hold one hand steady palmar side down and with the other hand tap the dorsum (back) of the steady hand first with the palmar aspect and then with the dorsal aspect of the fingers, repetitively pronating and supinating the forearm in the process. If there is a cerebellar problem the patient will be clumsy and there will be fluctuations in both speed and amplitude of the movement. This clinical sign is called dysdiadokokinesis.

Heel–shin test. With the patient sitting or lying ask the patient to place the heel of one foot on the shin of the opposite leg just below the knee. Then ask them to run the heel along the shin to the foot and bring it back to the knee. Cerebellar problems will be manifest by the wandering of the heel away from the intended path.

 PITFALL

These tests are difficult for the normal elderly to perform so you need to look for subtle differences between the two sides and also more than one positive sign

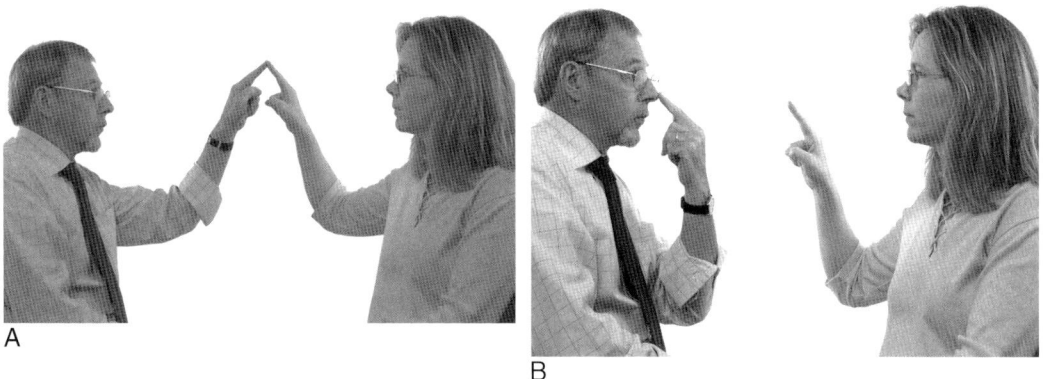

Fig. 11.9 Finger–nose test (reproduced with permission of BASICS Scotland).

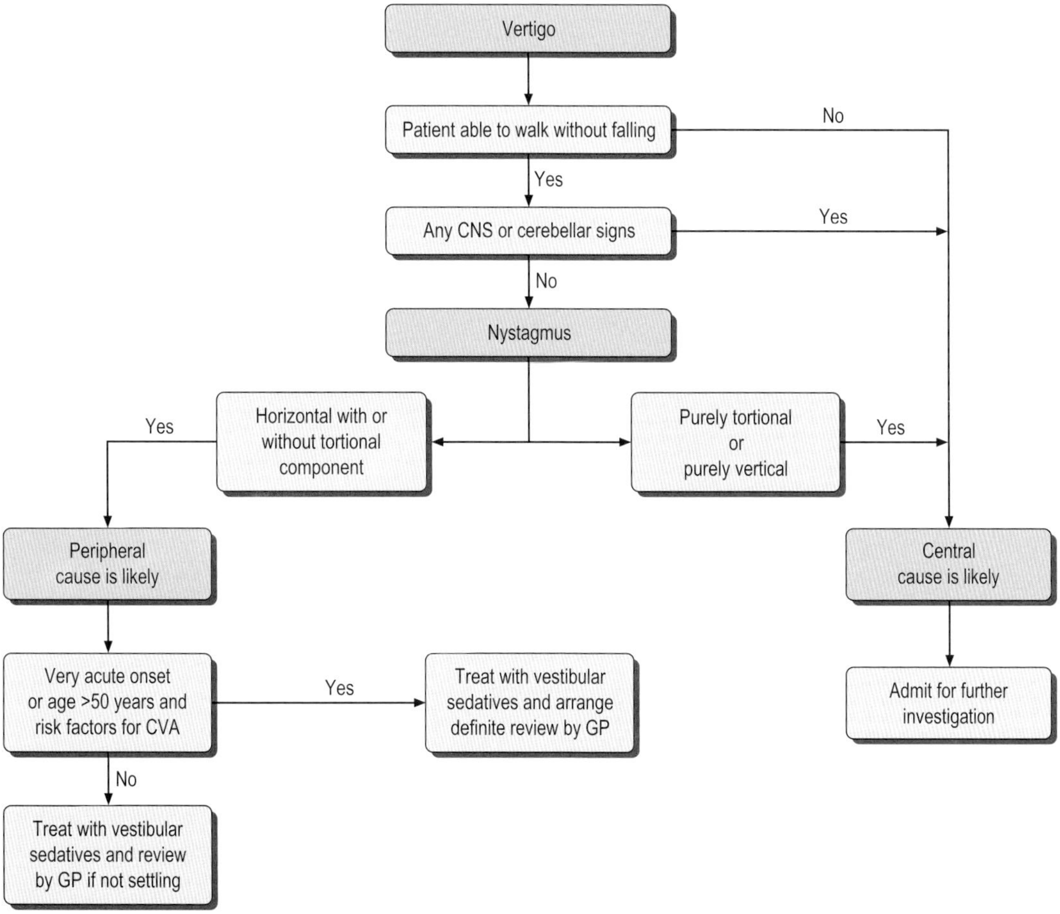

Vertigo

↓

Patient able to walk without falling —— No ——→

↓ Yes

Any CNS or cerebellar signs —— Yes ——→

↓ No

Nystagmus

Yes ←—— Horizontal with or without tortional component ←——→ Purely tortional or purely vertical —— Yes ——→

↓

Peripheral cause is likely

Central cause is likely

↓

Very acute onset or age >50 years and risk factors for CVA —— Yes ——→ Treat with vestibular sedatives and arrange definite review by GP

↓ No

Treat with vestibular sedatives and review by GP if not settling

Admit for further investigation

Fig. 11.10 Assessing the cause of vertigo.

Meniere's syndrome

Patients with Meniere's syndrome occasionally present with an isolated episode of severe vertigo that lasts for hours and is followed by a sensation of unsteadiness and dizziness for days. Typically, however, the vertigo is preceded or accompanied by reduced hearing, tinnitus that changes in pitch in association with the episode and a sense of fullness or blocking of the ear. Over time, the attacks of Meniere's syndrome recur, and fluctuations in hearing and episodes of tinnitus may be followed by a residual, low-frequency, sensorineural hearing loss. Fluctuating hearing levels associated with recurrent episodes of vertigo are central to the diagnosis of Meniere's syndrome. Examination of the ear may show deafness but ENT examination is otherwise normal and CNS examination is normal.

Vestibular neuronitis

Vestibular neuronitis is a clinical syndrome characterised by the acute onset of rotatory vertigo, which is associated with spontaneous nystagmus, postural imbalance and nausea without accompanying cochlear or neurological symptoms. It typically begins over a period of a few hours, peaks in the first day, and then improves within days. Disabling vertigo usually resolves within a week, but it may be followed by a sensation of unsteadiness or transient episodes of dizziness. Complete recovery from the symptoms usually occurs within weeks to months.

Benign paroxysmal positional vertigo

This is the commonest cause of vertigo. The classic symptoms include vertigo that appears with a few seconds latency when changing position of the head in space. The vertigo fades in 30–60 seconds. The dizziness is combined with a nystagmus beating in the direction of the affected canal. The condition is caused by debris in the semicircular canals.

Cerebrovascular event

Cerebellar TIAs or CVAs can present with vertigo. Symptoms are usually sudden onset and associated with nystagmus, ataxia and subtle co-ordination problems. Other neurological manifestations may or may not be present. Co-ordination can be assessed using the finger–nose test, hand tapping and heel–shin test. Hearing loss and tinnitus tend not to be features and examination of the ear is normal. Patients with an acute cerebellar stroke are often unable to walk without falling. Current recommendations are that all patients with suspected TIA or CVA are admitted to hospital for further investigation and treatment. However, unless the vertigo is particularly disabling or there are social reasons admission can be delayed if there is diagnostic uncertainty. If a decision is made not to admit, the patient will require to see a GP within 24 hours.

Other central causes usually present insidiously.

Facial pain

Facial pain can be associated with sinusitis, dental abscesses and many other less common conditions. Helpful questions in the history are:

■ do you have any problems with your teeth at present?
■ any trouble with your jaw when you eat?
■ do you have migraine headaches?
■ is the pain worse if you bend over?
■ history of a recent URTI?

Examination of the patient with facial pain should include inspection of the face for facial symmetry, erythema, blisters and swelling. Look in the mouth for pharyngitis, condition of teeth and any gum swelling or redness. Ask the patient to open and close the mouth, listen and feel for any jaw clicking. Palpate over the sinuses feeling for tenderness. Check the ears as described above.

Sinusitis

Sinusitis can be viral or bacterial. Sinusitis presents with facial pain, blocked nose, mucopurulent nasal discharge and anosmia (loss of sense of smell). Referred pain may be present in teeth and ears. Evidence-based treatment consists of simple analgesia/NSAID, reduction of congestion and antibiotic treatment – usually amoxicillin as first line.[10]

Dental abscess

Patients with a dental abscess often present with a unilateral swollen throbbing face. Treatment should be provided by a dental practitioner ASAP. However, advice regarding analgesia may be given.

Non-ENT causes of facial pain

Shingles may present with unilateral facial pain before the onset of blisters. Blisters associated with shingles are always unilateral. Patients should be advised to take simple analgesia and contact their own GP within 72 hours of the onset of any blisters (see Chapter 12). Trigeminal neuralgia can present with paroxysms of severe unilateral pain in the trigeminal nerve distribution lasting only seconds, separated by pain-free periods. The pain is often described as severe electric shocks. Contraction of the facial and masticatory muscles during an episode may occur. It should be treated with simple analgesia in the first instance and advice to see their GP.

Facial weakness (Bell's palsy)

Facial weakness affects both sexes equally but is commonest between the ages of 10 and 40 years. It presents as a weakness of the seventh cranial (facial) nerve, the nerve that controls movement of the muscles of the face, the stapedius muscle, taste sensation of the anterior two-thirds of the tongue and lacrimal gland secretory function. The cause is often not clear, although herpes infections may be involved. Pain behind or in front of the ear may precede weakness of facial muscles by 1–2 days. Loss of taste (anterior two-thirds of the tongue) and sensitivity to sound (hyperacusis) on the affected side may be present in greater than 50% of cases. Patients often complain of headache and that their face feels stiff or pulled to one side. Objectively they have difficulty with eating and drinking and a change in facial appearance with facial droop, difficulty with facial expressions, difficulty closing one eye, difficulty with fine facial movements, drooling due to inability to control facial muscles and dry eye secondary to being unable to close eye properly because of facial weakness.

Examination shows upper and lower facial weakness, which is almost always isolated to one side of the face or occasionally to the forehead, eyelid or mouth. Despite subjective sensory symptoms, the loss of sensation on examination is a rare and disturbing finding. If associated with a blistering rash typical of herpes zoster on ears or palate, Ramsey–Hunt syndrome should be suspected (see above). Presentations outwith the typical age groups, bilateral or polyneuropathies have a higher incidence of underlying causes and need investigation. All patients should be advised to see their GP for follow-up. If the patient presents out of hours they require reassurance that the majority of cases resolve within 3 weeks. There is no substantial evidence at present for the use of prednisolone or aciclovir in the treatment of Bell's palsy, although many people are still treated with medications based on results of non-randomised trials. There are currently ongoing randomised controlled clinical trials looking at the treatment of Bell's palsy.

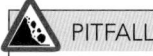 **PITFALL**

A cerebrovascular event is the commonest cause of facial weakness in the elderly

Sudden hearing loss

This is a rare presentation. Important points in the history are:

- is the hearing loss partial or complete?
- one side or both?
- has there been any noise exposure or trauma?

Examination may reveal wax impaction, a perforated tympanic membrane or a normal ear. If the ear looks normal a CNS examination is mandatory to look for other signs that would point to a cerebrovascular event as the cause of the hearing loss. Wax impaction is treated with softening drops and ear syringing several days later. Perforated tympanic membranes are treated as above. If a cerebrovascular event is suspected current recommendations support admission to hospital for investigation and treatment. However if there are no other symptoms or signs the patient should be referred to the GP for assessment.

Trauma (facial fractures)

Maxillofacial injury is rarely life-threatening unless it results in airway obstruction or severe blood loss. In both situations it is often associated with severe head and cervical spine injury. Many patients with more minor injuries will present the day following injury with swelling, bruising, closed eye and painful jaw. These patients will require a full assessment and usually referral to an A&E department, with imaging facilities. The exception is a suspected fractured nose. If this is the only injury the patient should be assessed for epistaxis, septal haematoma, and nasal obstruction. If none of these are present advice should be given regarding analgesia, not blowing or picking the nose, and to see their own GP for discussion on further management once swelling has subsided (usually around 7–10 days). If these symptoms are present referral to hospital for further assessment is required.

References

1 Cates C 1999 An evidence-based approach to reducing antibiotic use in children with acute otitis media: controlled before and after study. BMJ 318:715

2 Little P, Gould C, Williamson I et al 2001 Pragmatic randomised controlled trial of two prescribing strategies for childhood acute otitis media. BMJ 322:336–342

3 SIGN 2004 Diagnosis and management of childhood otitis media in primary care. Report No. 66. Scottish Intercollegiate Guidelines Network. Available online: http://www.sign.ac.uk/guidelines/fulltext/66/section3.html (5 Mar 2007)

4 Glasziou P P, Del Mar C B, Sanders S L, Hayem M 2003 Antibiotics for acute otitis media in children (Cochrane Review). The Cochrane Library (Issue 2). Update Software, Oxford

5 Takata G S, Chan L S, Shekelle P et al 2001 Evidence assessment of management of acute otitis media: 1. The role of antibiotics in treatment of uncomplicated acute otitis media. Pediatrics 108:239–247

6 Damoiseaux R A M J, van Balen F A M, Hoes A W et al 2000 Primary care based randomised, double blind trial of amoxicillin versus placebo for acute otitis media in children aged under 2 years. BMJ 320:350–354

7 NZGG 1998 Acute otitis media: meta-analysis. New Zealand Guidelines Group. Available online: http://www.nzgg.org.nz/index.cfm (5 Mar 2007)

8 American Academy of Pediatrics and American Academy of Family Physicians 2004 Diagnosis and management of acute otitis media. Pediatrics 113:1451–1465

9 Hotson J R, Baloh R W 1998 Acute vestibular syndrome. N Engl J Med 339:680–686

10 Del Mar C, Glasziou P 2003 Upper respiratory tract infection. Clin Evid 9:1701–1711

Management of allergy, rashes and itching

Introduction

The vast majority of skin problems that present in the community are minor in nature. Unfortunately, very occasionally, the development of seemingly innocuous symptoms such as a rash and/or itching can be the presenting symptoms of a life-threatening condition – namely anaphylaxis or meningococcal septicaemia. Whilst other clinical conditions can mimic both anaphylaxis and meningitis, especially in the early stages, there are usually clues in the presentation that help to minimise the delays in administering appropriate therapy. It is not possible in this chapter to cover all potential causes of a skin rash and/or itching. Rather, this chapter aims to focus on important conditions that require recognition, treatment and possible referral in the acute pre-hospital setting. The objectives of this chapter are listed in Box 12.1.

BOX 12.1 Chapter objectives

With regard to the presentation of a rash and/or itching:
- To understand the basic physiology and pathology underlying allergic causes of rashes and itching
- To perform a primary survey of the patient and treat any immediately life-threatening problems
- To identify any patients who have a normal primary survey but have an obvious need for hospital admission
- To perform a secondary survey incorporating other body systems that may be affected by a skin rash and/or itching
- To consider a list of differential diagnoses
- Discuss treatment based on the likely diagnosis(es)
- Discuss appropriate patient follow-up
- Describe who can be safely considered for home treatment

Basic physiology and pathology

Allergic reactions are linked to the release of chemical mediators, which are released from mast cells in a process known as degranulation.[1] This occurs when an allergen cross links with immunoglobulin E (IgE) bound to receptors on mast cells. These chemicals are either released immediately (immediate allergic reaction), or after a few hours (late phase response) (Table 12.1). This timing helps to guide appropriate treatment.

TABLE 12.1 Release of chemical mediators from mast cells		
Timing of release	Examples	Treatment
Immediate	Histamine, tryptase, hydrolases	Anti-histamines (e.g. chlorpheniramine, cetirizine)
Delayed	Prostaglandins, leukotrienes, cytokines	Steroids (e.g. prednisolone)

Primary survey

Assess for an ABC problem in patients with itching and/or a rash (Box 12.2). The recognition of developing airway obstruction is critical, particularly in the presence of anaphylaxis. Patients may complain initially of a feeling of tightening in the throat, be unable to complete sentences or have audible airway noise (stridor or wheeze). If airway obstruction becomes complete, then prompt initiation of a surgical airway will be required.

BOX 12.2 Primary survey
Arrange immediate treatment and transfer to hospital if any of the following are present: ■ Signs of airway obstruction ■ Respiratory rate <10 or >29 ■ Oxygen saturation <92% on air ■ Pulse rate <50 or >120 ■ Systolic BP <90 ■ GCS <12

Patients with a normal primary survey with obvious need for hospital admission

The following conditions may present initially with a normal primary survey but immediate treatment (if appropriate) and hospital admission should be initiated:

■ Suspected rash of meningococcal septicaemia
■ Definite exposure to a trigger that has previously led to an anaphylactic reaction

- Self-administration of epinephrine by a patient for a suspected anaphylactic reaction
- A suspected anaphylactic reaction that has not fully developed
- Cellulitis – patient clinically toxic or affecting the peri-orbital tissues.

The history and findings on examination should help to establish whether you are faced with such a scenario. Although these patients may not have abnormal clinical signs at the time of assessment, this should not lull you into a false sense of security since they may deteriorate rapidly. In the case of suspected meningococcal septicaemia, early administration of appropriate antibiotic therapy is safe and associated with an improved prognosis.[2] Whenever there is a suspicion of anaphylaxis, epinephrine for intramuscular injection should be readily available.[3] If the above situations present, based on the history and examination findings as described in this chapter, then appropriate treatment should be administered and hospital admission arranged.

Secondary survey (including history taking)

Having ensured that your patient has no immediately life-threatening problems on their primary survey or the need for immediate hospital admission, you will be left with a patient for whom a careful history and examination should elucidate whether further treatment is required and whether or not the patient can be safely left at home. A history of the presenting complaint should be taken, any other information noted and an examination performed as described earlier in this series. Remember that the skin is the largest organ in the body and adequate exposure may be required to allow a thorough examination to be completed. Obviously, the degree of exposure will be dictated by the prevailing circumstances and nature of the presenting complaint(s).

History

The following will be helpful in establishing the diagnosis in someone presenting with a rash or itching. Unfortunately, there are few clinical tests that can help in the diagnostic process, which relies heavily on the use of a logical process to identify and eliminate serious problems.

Onset of symptoms

Did the symptoms come on suddenly over the course of a few minutes/hours or more gradually over the course of several days? Has there been recent injury to the area affected (especially a laceration)? Can symptoms be related to a particular event? In particular, the patient may be able to

PITFALL

Nuts are increasingly being used as a 'filler' in a wide range of foods – the patient may not therefore be aware that they have consumed nut products

associate the symptoms with a specific trigger, e.g. consumption of a particular meal, use of a new shampoo, etc. The common potential triggers for an anaphylactic reaction are listed in Table 12.2.

TABLE 12.2 Potential triggers for anaphylaxis	
Cause	Examples
Foods	Nuts and seeds, eggs, seafood, kiwi fruit, bananas
Venom/stings	Bees, wasps, jellyfish, ants, snakebites
Drugs	Antibiotics, aspirin/NSAIDs*, vaccines, radio contrast dye
Physical contacts	Latex rubber
Other	Cold temperatures, exercise

*Non-steroidal anti-inflammatory drugs (e.g. ibuprofen, diclofenac, naproxen, etc.)

Rash/swelling

If a rash is present then is it localised or generalised? What colour is the rash? Does the area of the rash itself itch or is it actually painful to touch? Does the rash change colour when pressed against the edge of a glass? If swelling is present, which part(s) of the body are affected? Pay particular heed to any swelling involving the mouth, tongue or eyes.

Associated symptoms

Of utmost importance is whether the patient feels generally well in him/herself. Does the patient have a generalised itch all over? Is there disturbance of another bodily system – e.g. gastrointestinal upset? Specific enquiry should be made about the presence of vomiting, headache, neck pain, cough and eye discomfort. The patient should be asked whether they have recently had an upper respiratory tract infection and/or tonsillitis.

Progress of symptoms

It is important to ascertain whether the symptoms have continued to worsen since their onset. Anaphylaxis and meningococcal septicaemia are progressive conditions that will steadily deteriorate with time. However, if a patient with an allergic reaction but without signs of anaphylaxis has remained stable for more than an hour they are unlikely to deteriorate further.

Previous episodes

Ask whether a similar episode has affected the patient before. Previous episodes of anaphylaxis are unlikely to be easily forgotten! Unfortunately, a history of a previous allergic reaction (mild or severe) does not predict the likelihood of an anaphylactic reaction – a reaction can still occur despite a long history of previous safe exposure.[4]

Risk factors

Exposure to certain triggers is associated with an increased incidence of allergic reactions (Table 12.2).

Past medical history/drug history

Any past history of similar events should be noted. Many drugs can be implicated in the development of allergic reactions and anaphylaxis. Aspirin accounts for about 3% of anaphylactic reactions and symptoms may occur hours after ingestion.[5] Those allergic to aspirin may also be sensitive to NSAIDs, which may cause a similar reaction. A similar allergic relationship can occur with penicillins and cephalosporins. Even people who have had no previous problems with penicillins may experience an anaphylactoid reaction after taking them. Diabetics are at a higher risk of cellulitis.

Family and social history

A positive family history of similar episodes suggests hereditary angio-neurotic oedema (HANE), which is inherited as an autosomal dominant trait. Has the patient been in contact with anyone who has had similar symptoms or felt unwell? Is the patient worried about a particular diagnosis? If so, this should be excluded if possible so that the patient may be reassured.

Examination

See Chapter 2 relating to patient examination. It is always advisable to check and document the vital signs of any patient who presents with a possible allergic reaction or rash. This includes the measurement of temperature, pulse, blood pressure and respiratory rate. An elevated temperature and/or the presence of enlarged (and often painful) lymph glands in the submandibular and/or cervical regions suggests the possibility of an infective process. It is sensible to test for neck stiffness in any patient who presents with a rash and systemic upset. The patient's neck should be passively flexed forwards towards the chest wall, a manoeuvre that should not be painful to complete. If neck flexion causes pain, then Kernig's and Brudzinski's signs should be tested:

- Kernig's sign. Extend the knee with the hip flexed – positive test if hamstrings contraction occurs as a result
- Brudzinski's sign. Flex the neck passively – test is positive if the knees and hips flex as a result.

PITFALL

Although a positive response to Kernig's or Brudzinski's tests is diagnostic of meningism, the *absence* of a positive response does *not* rule out meningitis

General examination

Note the patient's overall demeanour. Do they appear well, at ease and able to converse normally or are they anxious, sweaty, confused or making abnormal noises as they breathe? If this is the case, go back and reassess their primary survey and consider whether further treatment and/or onward referral are required.

Examination of the skin

PITFALL

Although a non-blanching purpuric rash should be considered to be indicative of meningococcal septicaemia in the pre-hospital setting, neither the *absence* of a rash nor the fact that a rash blanches should be considered as ruling out meningitis or septicaemia

As previously mentioned, it is important to ensure adequate exposure of the skin, especially in younger children who may be less able or likely to bring the presence of a rash to your attention. In a significant proportion of patients with meningococcal septicaemia, the rash starts on the palms of the hands and/or the soles of the feet so be sure to examine these carefully. Is the rash painful to the touch? Document any swelling of the tissues, especially around the face and the eyes. Gently examine inside the mouth looking for swelling of the tongue. Note the presence of any scratch marks on the body. Note the colour associated with any rash – does the rash disappear or change colour when pressure is applied? (Ideally this should be done with the base of a clear glass.) Table 12.3 lists the common terms used to describe physical changes in the skin associated with the presence of a rash.

Investigations

There are few investigations that will quickly confirm the diagnosis of a rash or itching in the acute pre-hospital setting. The diagnosis usually requires a clinical interpretation of the symptoms and signs presented.

Differential diagnosis

Table 12.4 lists the main important conditions to be distinguished in a patient presenting with a rash and/or itching. Further information is given later in this chapter specific to each condition.

TABLE 12.3 Terms used to describe rash-induced skin changes

Terminology	Description	Clinical examples
Macular	Non-infiltrated flat lesions which differ in colour from adjacent areas of skin	Erythema, purpura
Papular	Well demarcated raised lesions in the skin of varying sizes	Urticarial wheals, planar warts
Vesicular	Small protuberances with a central cavity containing clear liquid	Chickenpox
Excoriations	Very superficial wounds in the surface of the skin	Scratches
Purpura	Small patches of non-blanching discolouration caused by bleeding from small superficial blood vessels in the skin Petechiae – Small spots of purpura Ecchymoses – Large confluent patches of purpura	Meningococcal disease Idiopathic thrombocytopaenic purpura (ITP) Henoch–Schonlein purpura (HSP)

TABLE 12.4 Conditions presenting with rash and/or itch or itch alone

Rash ± itch	Itching alone
Immune system mediated Anaphylaxis Anaphylactoid reaction Allergic reaction – local Urticaria ('hives') and/or angioedema Idiopathic thrombocytopaenic purpura (ITP)	**Immune system mediated** Anaphylaxis Anaphylactoid reaction
Infective *a. Bacterial* Meningococcal septicaemia Cellulitis Impetigo Scarlet fever	**Systemic** Systemic upset (e.g. uraemia, cholestasis, blood disorders)
b. Viral Varicella zoster Primary infection (chickenpox) Reactivation (herpes zoster or 'shingles') Measles Rubella (German measles) Non-specific viral rash	**Other** Senile itch Solid tumours HIV
c. Other conditions Henoch–Schonlein purpura Psoriasis Eczema	

Management plan

Depending on the suspected diagnosis and clinical condition of the patient, the usual management plan can be summarised as one of the following five choices:

■ Group 1 – Features requiring hospital referral. Examples would be an unwell child with a suspected meningococcal rash, an anaphylactic reaction.
■ Group 2 – Patients who need a disease 'rule-out'. These are borderline cases with some features of a diagnosis but the clinical picture is not sufficiently clear to make a definite decision on management. They need further investigation and possibly further observation. Examples would be a petechial rash in a well child. These cases may need to be referred to A&E or to the appropriate inpatient team.
■ Group 3 – Common features allowing diagnosis of a problem which may be treated at home. Examples would include a young man with urticaria and no features of anaphylaxis or scabies.
■ Group 4 – Type of patient who may be treated by a wait-and-see approach. This group has no specific symptoms or signs that indicate serious pathology at the time of assessment. These patients may be managed at home with advice that the diagnosis is not clear but *at present* there are no signs of serious pathology. The patient should be advised to seek further advice if symptoms fail to settle or get worse.
■ Group 5 – Social implications. Some patients may need referral, such as the very elderly or very young, due to difficulty coping at home as well as the tendency for more rapid deterioration in condition.

Where indicated, appropriate home management options are discussed for each condition.

Immune system mediated conditions

Anaphylaxis and anaphylactoid reactions

■ Management group 1 – admit and treat immediately

Anaphylaxis refers to a severe generalised allergic reaction, whereby specific triggers (e.g. insect stings, peanuts) stimulate the release of IgE immunoglobulin. This IgE release causes vasodilation, airway swelling and capillary leakage leading to hypotension. An anaphylactoid reaction results in an identical situation, but does not involve the release of IgE. An example of this is the reaction that can be seen to radiography dye.[6] Whilst no universally accepted definition exists, a good working definition is 'a severe allergic reaction to any stimulus, (usually) having sudden onset and generally lasting less than 24 hours, involving one or more body systems and producing one or more symptoms such as hives, flushing, itching, angio-oedema, stridor, wheezing, shortness of breath, vomiting, diarrhoea or shock'.[7] The rate of anaphylaxis in the UK has risen from 6 per million in 1990/91 to 41 per million in 2000/01.[8]

Symptoms and signs of anaphylaxis

The diagnosis of anaphylaxis is clinical. Symptoms usually begin within minutes of exposure to the trigger(s), but may be delayed by several hours. Many of the symptoms and signs of anaphylaxis may mimic other clinical conditions, thus leading to a delay in diagnosis (Table 12.5). For this reason, the first attack is particularly dangerous. Having experienced the symptoms once, a surviving patient is likely to recognise their occurrence in the future thus aiding earlier diagnosis and treatment. Over 90% of patients with anaphylaxis will develop cutaneous symptoms such as urticaria (see later), itching and angio-oedema that can help to distinguish the condition from other diagnoses. A vasovagal reaction, perhaps the commonest mimic of an anaphylactic episode, does not involve cutaneous changes, tachycardia or bronchospasm. Patients often describe a non-specific but frightening feeling of 'impending doom'.

TABLE 12.5 Differential diagnosis of anaphylaxis

Symptom/signs of anaphylaxis	Differential diagnosis(es)
Respiratory compromise (shortness of breath, wheeze, stridor)	Asthma, COPD, inhaled foreign body, pulmonary embolism
Loss of consciousness (LOC)	Vasovagal reaction, seizures, cardiac event (e.g. arrhythmia)
Hypotension	Vasovagal reaction, shock (cardiogenic/septic/hypovolaemic)
Collapse	As for hypotension/LOC plus panic attack, hyperventilation syndrome, Munchausen's syndrome
Cutaneous skin flushing	Vasovagal reaction, carcinoid syndrome, postmenopausal flushing
Gastrointestinal (diarrhoea, abdominal cramps, nausea and vomiting)	Hereditary angio-neurotic oedema (HANE), food poisoning

Untreated, anaphylaxis will steadily worsen and a progressive deterioration in the patient's clinical condition should alert an observer to the possibility of this diagnosis. Patients with significant cardiovascular collapse may be unable to give a coherent history, adding to the potential for diagnostic delay.

Management of anaphylaxis

The management of suspected anaphylaxis is a medical emergency. Early recognition of symptoms, removal of the triggering source (if possible) and prompt administration of epinephrine (adrenaline) are the fundamentals of successful management.

ABCs

Airway patency must be maintained and 100% oxygen should be applied to all patients as soon as it is available. If the patient has developed signs of complete airway obstruction then a surgical airway must be initiated. Intravenous access should be established as large volumes of fluid may be required to treat the severe hypotension often seen in anaphylaxis, if it does not correct rapidly with drug treatment. A rapid infusion of 1–2 litres of crystalloid or colloid, given in 250–500 ml boluses, may be required if the radial pulse is lost. Children should receive an initial bolus of 20 ml/kg with boluses repeated until a response is noted.

Epinephrine

Epinephrine (adrenaline) 0.5 mg (0.5 ml of 1:1000) should be injected intramuscularly, preferably into the antero-lateral aspect of the upper arm or thigh. This route of administration has been shown to be superior to subcutaneous injection.[9] Epinephrine should be re-administered every 5 minutes until clinical improvement occurs. Individuals taking beta-blockers may have a suboptimal response to epinephrine, with possible persistent severe hypotension and bradycardia.[10] The latter can be treated with atropine (0.3–0.5 mg IM every 10 minutes to a maximum of 2 mg). Glucagon (as a 1 mg IV bolus) may also be effective for patients taking beta-blockers although it is not licensed for this indication.[6,10]

Anti-histamines

Histamine is one of the prime chemical mediators of the anaphylactic reaction. Anti-histamine drugs may therefore provide rapid relief of distressing symptoms. A H_1 antagonist drug such as chlorpheniramine (10–20 mg IM or slow IV) may be combined with a H_2 antagonist such as ranitidine (150 mg orally, if able to take) to effect maximal histamine blockade.[11]

PITFALL

Rapid administration of intravenous chlorpheniramine or steroids can cause hypotension

PITFALL

Bronchospasm should improve with the administration of a beta-2 agonist, but this does not mean that the anaphylactic process is resolving or that epinephrine is not required

Corticosteroids

Corticosteroids, in the form of hydrocortisone 200 mg (IV or IM) or prednisolone (oral) 50 mg should be administered to minimise the likelihood and severity of second-phase reactions. The benefits of administering steroids can take 6–12 hours to be realised, and it is emphasised that their main therapeutic influence is upon recurrent or protracted episodes. Even so, it is recognised that patients who have received steroids may still develop severe biphasic or prolonged reactions.[12,13]

Beta-2 agonists

Bronchospasm is often a prominent symptom of anaphylaxis and commonly manifests itself as shortness of breath and/or wheezing. It should be treated with a beta-2 agonist such as salbutamol (Ventolin) or terbutaline (Bricanyl). Depending on resources available, these may be administered via a standard inhaler device or through a nebuliser (oxygen-driven if possible). Beta-2 agonist therapy can be repeated as required or given continuously en route to hospital according to the degree of response achieved.

Admission to hospital

Although most episodes of anaphylaxis will occur and recover within 1–8 hours, the potential for a second-phase reaction remains. As a consequence, all patients who have sustained an anaphylactic reaction should be observed and monitored in a hospital setting. Local hospital policies may vary, but second-phase reactions can occur up to 24 hours after the initial episode, regardless of the response to treatment.[10,14] For the next 48 hours after discharge, it is recommended that the patient remain in an environment that permits easy access to medical attention should symptoms recur. This has important implications for those patients who live in isolated rural communities.

Follow-up arrangements

Following an episode of anaphylaxis, there are two important issues to address with the patient. Firstly, an attempt should be made to identify the precipitating cause and reduce the likelihood of further exposure. The likely cause may be obvious from the original clinical presentation or otherwise confirmation requires referral to an allergist for a skin prick test. Those who subsequently have a confirmed IgE-mediated allergy may be amenable to specific and potentially curative immunotherapy. Secondly, patients need to be aware of the correct actions in the event of a recurrence. They should be prescribed a self-injection device for the administration of epinephrine (e.g. Epi-Pen), be instructed in its appropriate use and advised to obtain a Medic-Alert bracelet or necklace. Close relatives, friends and/or neighbours should also be considered for education as deemed appropriate to the individual circumstance.

Allergic reactions – local

A far more common occurrence than anaphylaxis is the development of a localised reaction to an allergen without the development of serious generalised symptoms. The reaction seen after an insect bite is a classic example of this. There is usually (but not always) a history of exposure to a potential allergen, following which the patient may notice the development of skin changes such as rash, itching, swelling and/or pain. If the affected area involves the mouth or neck then the potential for airway compromise must be considered. There are three simple but important differentiations to be made which help to distinguish these less serious local reactions from those that may lead to a patient's deterioration:

■ the patient's symptoms are generally localised to the affected area
■ the patient has no symptoms or signs of systemic upset
■ the patient's symptoms do not progressively worsen.

Treatment

Simple measures such as the application of ice may help with swelling and pain. The use of an oral antihistamine such as cetirizine (which can be bought over the counter by the patient and used in patients from the age of 2 upwards) will alleviate most of the patient's symptoms within 1–3 days. If the reaction is more severe, then a 3-day course of oral steroids, e.g. prednisolone EC (1 mg/kg/day for children, 30 mg/day for adults), may be administered to help reduce the reaction. The patient should be advised to seek medical attention again if their symptoms worsen, become generalised or have not resolved after 3 days.

Urticaria ('hives') and angioedema

■ Management group 3 – home management if no features of concern

Urticaria and angioedema are related conditions and occur together in about 50% of cases, with urticaria a single entity in 40% and the remaining 10% being angioedema alone. The British Association of Dermatologists offers useful online information for both patients and doctors.[15]

Simple urticaria

This condition typically produces an itchy 'wheal and flare' reaction anywhere on the body. The lesions usually have a raised central area and blanch on direct pressure.

Angioedema and urticaria

This condition, which is more common in females, tends to affect the extremities (e.g. lips, eyelids and digits) and is often painful rather than itchy. The majority of episodes are acute and self-limiting but up to 10% will become chronic in nature. In the majority of cases, no definite causal agent is found although any of the substances in Table 12.1 may be implicated in some cases. The majority of symptoms will settle by 6 weeks and the patient can be reassured about the benign nature of the condition. Treatment in the acute phase involves avoidance of any obvious trigger(s) and the use of an oral H_1 antihistamine agent such as chlorpheniramine or cetirizine. In the event that one agent is ineffective, another should be substituted.[16] In the longer term, other agents including oral steroids may be required if the condition becomes chronic.

Angioedema without urticaria

The commonest cause of isolated angioedema is hereditary angio-neurotic oedema (HANE). This condition is characterised by recurrent acute swelling affecting the cutaneous tissues and mucous membranes of any part of the body. Most patients inherit the condition as an autosomal dominant gene and experience their first episode in childhood. The defect is a lack of C'1 esterase inhibitor protein which leads to inappropriate activation of the complement pathway. Triggers may include allergens but a reaction can also occur following fright or physical trauma. Patients are usually familiar with the pattern of their symptoms, which makes the diagnosis easier as their experience grows. Although the symptoms of swelling usually develop gradually over many hours, involvement of the upper airway tissues can cause concern. Management of an acute episode depends on its severity. Whilst peripheral swelling does not require active treatment, airway involvement requires active management including the administration of C'1 inhibitor concentrate.[17] Some patients may carry an auto-injector containing this drug, which should be administered immediately if available. Otherwise, urgent transfer to an alerted hospital is indicated.

Other causes of isolated angioedema may be linked to the use of certain medications (ACE inhibitors in particular). Angiotension-2 receptor antagonists (e.g. losartan) can be substituted as these are not associated with the condition. If no cause can be identified, the condition is deemed to be idiopathic.

Idiopathic thrombocytopaenic purpura (ITP)

■ Management group 2 – seek further advice from hospital

This is a condition where the body's immune system attacks platelets, the blood cells that help form blood clots. This leads to a low platelet count in the blood (detected through a full blood count). As a result, ITP causes small amounts of bleeding into the skin tissues. Its cause is unknown, but there are two forms – one that affects children (usually between 2–4 years old and frequently after a viral infection) and one that affects adults (usually women). It results in a non-blanching purpuric rash, sometimes with more extensive patches of bruising, but is not acutely life-threatening. Usually, individuals with ITP show no other signs of illness other than their rash – in contrast to patients with meningococcal disease. If in doubt as to the cause of purpura in the pre-hospital setting, further medical advice should be obtained or hospital admission arranged.

Infective conditions

Bacterial

Meningococcal septicaemia

- Management group 1 – admit and treat immediately

Meningococcal septicaemia is a life-threatening condition with high morbidity and mortality. In 2005, 721 cases were reported in England and Wales.[18] Unfortunately, particularly in its early stages, its symptoms are fairly non-specific and may mimic those of a common viral illness. Although it may not occur at all, the development of a rash is an important clinical sign, especially in the presence of systemic upset (e.g. headache, vomiting and/or altered mental status). The Meningitis Research Foundation (www.meningitis.org.uk) is one of many resources with practical advice and information for health professionals.

The classical rash of meningococcal septicaemia may consist of any of the following:

- tiny red or brown pin-prick marks (petechiae)
- purple blotches
- blood blisters.

The rash is usually described as 'non-blanching' – i.e. if a glass tumbler is pressed firmly against a septicaemic rash, the marks will not fade. In its initial phase, the rash may not have any of the classical features described. In the case of any patient with a rash, the patient and/or their carers should be educated about features of possible concern and advised to seek advice again if the nature of the rash changes. It often starts first on the sole of the feet or the palm of the hands. The rash may not be as distinct in patients with darkly coloured skin, in whom areas such as the conjunctiva and the roof of the mouth should be checked carefully. Patients with septicaemia will usually become seriously ill, often within a short time frame. Symptoms may be very subtle in infants and may include irritability, poor feeding, weak cry and mottled skin. If in doubt, the infant should be admitted for observation. In the case of suspected meningococcal septicaemia, appropriate antibiotic treatment should be administered as soon as possible. Pre-hospital antibiotic administration has been shown to reduce the mortality in meningococcal meningitis by approximately 50%. The incidence of true anaphylactic reactions to penicillin is extremely low and treatment should not be delayed unless there is a clear personal history of such.[19] In these circumstances, ceftriaxone is the preferred alternative.[20] The recommended doses of each drug are given in Table 12.6.

TABLE 12.6 Recommended dosages of antibiotics in the treatment of meningococcal septicaemia		
Patient's age	Penicillin V	Ceftriaxone
Infant	300 mg	100 mg/kg
Child (1–9 years)	600 mg	100 mg/kg
Child (10+ years)	1.2 g	1 g
Adult (16+ years)	1.2 g	1 g

Cellulitis

- Management group 2 (admit semi-urgently) or 3 (treat at home) – depending on severity

Cellulitis is an acute bacterial infection of the skin and subcutaneous tissues. Most commonly it involves the lower leg although any part of the body may be affected. Untreated, infection can spread and lead to septicaemia. Cellulitis involving the peri-orbital or orbital areas is of particular concern as infection may spread to the sagittal sinuses. The commonest clinical sign initially is a hot, raised and erythematous area of skin which is tender to the touch. As the cellulitis develops, the patient may develop systemic signs of infection (raised temperature, sweats, tachycardia and a feeling of malaise). The usual organisms involved are haemolytic streptococci and *Staphylococcus aureus*.[21] The history may indicate the portal of entry for the bacteria such as a laceration, abrasion or recent surgery. The mainstay of treatment is a combination of antibiotic therapy, analgesia, elevation of affected limbs and treatment of any underlying condition.

Antibiotic therapy

The standard antibiotic combination for cellulitis is benzyl penicillin and flucloxacillin (both 500 mg 6-hourly for adults – see the BNF or

MIMS for paediatric dosing). An alternative for those hypersensitive to penicillin is erythromycin 500 mg 6-hourly. Hospital admission for intravenous antibiotics is recommended for patients with involvement of the (peri)orbital tissues, systemic symptoms and those unable to tolerate oral treatment.

Analgesia

Cellulitis is often painful. Adequate analgesia should be prescribed and the patient advised on minimising friction pain from clothes touching the affected area.

Elevation

An important aspect of management is to keep the affected limb elevated whenever possible. This helps to reduce tissue swelling and pain. Ideally the affected limb should be kept higher than the heart and gentle exercises promoted to encourage fluid movement and reduce the incidence of complications such as DVT and pressure ulceration.

Treatment of the underlying condition

Any obvious wound which may have acted as a portal of entry should be examined and treated appropriately. Embedded foreign bodies should be removed. Other predisposing factors include diabetes, pre-existing oedema or skin ulceration and vascular disease. Cellulitis resulting from a human or animal bite can involve multiple organisms. Wounds should be thoroughly cleaned and a wide spectrum antibiotic such as co-amoxiclav prescribed.

Impetigo

■ Management group 3 – treat at home

Impetigo is a highly contagious bacterial infection of the superficial tissues of the skin. It is spread by direct contact and is common amongst children. The most frequently implicated organisms are *Staphylococcus aureus* and group A beta-haemolytic streptococcus. Although healthy skin can be affected, these bacteria usually enter the skin through a cut, scratch or abrasion. The nose and peri-oral regions, being susceptible to minor trauma, are the usual sites of presentation. A red sore that oozes fluid or pus usually heralds the start of the infection. As the infection spreads, other lesions appear nearby which may be painful or itchy. The patient does not usually have a temperature but there may be swelling of the lymph glands nearby. Treatment has traditionally been with either topical or oral antibiotics. A recent meta-analysis highlighted the lack of a quality evidence base for the most effective treatment for impetigo.[22] The authors concluded that the use of a topical antibiotic (such as mupirocin [Bactroban] or fucidic acid [Fucidin]) for 7 days should be recommended in a patient with limited disease and no systemic upset.[22]

Oral antibiotics are reserved for more severe infections. The agents of choice are cephalexin, co-amoxiclav or erythromycin – all available in suspension form.[23]

Scarlet fever

■ Management group 4 – treat at home

This condition is associated with a bacterial infection of the throat caused by group A beta-haemolytic streptococcus. It usually occurs in children under the age of 18. Symptoms include a sore throat, fever, swollen cervical glands and a rash which usually lasts 2–5 days. This initially appears as tiny red bumps on the chest and abdomen before spreading all over the body. It has an appearance like sunburn with a rough feel. The diagnosis is confirmed by a throat swab, but treatment in the form of antibiotics (penicillin or erythromycin) is usually commenced on clinical grounds. Left untreated, complications such as nephritis or rheumatic fever can result.

Viral

■ Management group 3 – treat at home

A rash is a clinical feature of many viral infections. Most are self-limiting and require no specific treatments other than those aimed at reducing the associated symptoms, especially fever and itch. Some of the commoner infections to present (often with a rash) in the community are described in more detail below. Measles and rubella are notifiable diseases in the UK under the Public Health (Infectious Diseases) Regulations 1988; chickenpox is notifiable in Scotland only.

Varicella zoster – chickenpox and shingles

Varicella zoster presents as two clinical entities. Primary infection results in the rash known as chickenpox, a highly contagious illness, usually occurring in childhood outbreaks. The virus then lies dormant in nerve cells but may reactivate to cause herpes zoster, also known as 'shingles'. The risk of developing shingles increases with age and reduced immunocompetence (e.g. immunosuppressive drugs, HIV infection, cancer).[24]

Chickenpox (notifiable in Scotland)

In Scotland in 2001 there were 21 894 notifications of chickenpox (428 per 100 000 population). The classic symptoms of chickenpox are a rash, fever and the general feeling of malaise seen with other viral infections. The rash usually appears within 2 weeks of exposure to the virus, with superficial spots that soon develop into blisters that burst and crust over. It is often intensely itchy and (a diagnostic pointer) spreads above the face and into the hair line. The rash remains a source of infection until all the blisters have crusted over. Chickenpox can spread to any individual who has not been previously infected or vaccinated. Although in childhood it is usually a mild illness, it can lead to complications including cellulitis, pneumonia and encephalitis.

Chickenpox can also cause problems in pregnancy – mothers who have no immunity should avoid contact with individuals with the illness and seek urgent medical advice if contact has taken place. Specific immunoglobulin can be administered to reduce the likelihood of subsequent infection. In the absence of any complications, treatment is symptomatic and should focus on standard drugs for fever reduction, and anti-histamines for associated itch. The affected individual should be isolated from contact with the general public and family members with no personal history of chickenpox until the rash has completely crusted over.

Shingles

Initially, patients with shingles usually experience a non-specific prodrome similar to that of other viral infections, followed by an area of abnormal skin sensation which may last 1–5 days before the appearance of the rash. Clusters of vesicles then appear which ultimately may ulcerate before crusting. The rash never crosses the midline and follows the line of one or more dermatomes. Pain of varying severity is present in virtually all patients. The rash heals in 2–4 weeks but may leave areas of scarring and altered pigmentation. In the acute phase, treatment involves the administration of appropriate analgesia. Initially this may take the form of paracetamol, with or without codeine (cocodamol). Resistant cases may require the use of adjuvant pain relief such as amitriptyline, gabapentin or carbamazepine. Antiviral therapy in the form of aciclovir, valaciclovir or famciclovir should be targeted towards those with the highest risk of complications – the immunocompromised, the elderly, those with a large surface area involved and those in severe pain at presentation. Use of these agents also reduces the incidence and severity of post herpetic neuralgia (PHN) – defined as pain that persists more than 30 days after the onset of the rash.

The incidence of PHN increases with age. Patients with a shingles rash on the forehead, around the eye or the nose have a 50% risk of developing severe eye complications. All such individuals should be referred to an eye specialist immediately for assessment.

Measles (notifiable)

Measles is the most frequent cause of vaccine-preventable deaths in childhood.[25] It is primarily a viral respiratory tract infection, which can have serious or even fatal consequences for infants and small children. In 2003, there were 2488 cases notified to the Health Protection

Agency.[18] Protection is currently offered through the MMR vaccination. Unfortunately, since a link between this vaccine and the development of autism was suggested in 1998,[26] reduced public confidence has resulted in a decreased uptake in vaccination, heralding the possibility of a major measles outbreak. Whilst subsequent studies have conclusively shown no association and some of the authors of the original study have also conceded that MMR has no causal role,[27] vaccine uptake remains as low as 61% in the UK.

Measles usually begins with a fever, a persistent cough, runny nose and sore throat. Two or three days later, the characteristic Koplik's spots appear. These are tiny red spots on the inner mucosal lining of the cheek. Subsequently, the fever increases and a more generalised red blotchy rash develops on the face, along the hairline and behind the ears. This slightly itchy rash rapidly spreads downward to the chest and back and, finally, to the thighs and feet. The rash tends to fade within 7 days with the illness itself lasting 10–14 days. Measles is infectious from about 4 days before to 4 days after the rash appears. Complications include ear infections, pneumonia, encephalitis and diarrhoea/vomiting. Non-immune pregnant women should seek specialist advice. Treatment is again largely symptomatic, and involves isolating the individual from the general public and susceptible family members.

Rubella – German measles (notifiable)

Although caused by a different virus, rubella shares some characteristics with measles (hence its synonym – 'germanus' being Latin for similar). Rubella is neither as contagious nor as serious as measles, except that it can have serious consequences for the unborn child of an unprotected mother. Protection is again provided by the MMR vaccine which has dramatically reduced the incidence of the condition. General symptoms, although milder, tend to be similar to measles but rarely last longer than 3 days. A fine, pink rash usually begins on the face and quickly spreads to the trunk and then the arms and legs before disappearing. Aching joints may occur, as may tender enlargement of the cervical lymph nodes. Rubella very rarely causes complications outwith pregnancy, where infection in the first trimester can lead to congenital abnormalities developing in up to 90% of cases. Symptomatic treatment and isolation are the only usual requirements for rubella.

Non-specific viral rashes

Virtually any viral infection can result in the development of a rash, usually on the face, chest or back. The rash is usually very fine, red in colour and blanches on pressure. It usually appears several days into the illness, often around the time the fever and other symptoms are improving. It may itch slightly but should not be painful. Care should be taken to exclude more serious causes of rashes (as outlined above). The individual affected may have symptoms such as a sore throat, runny nose, cough or lethargy but has no symptoms of concern. The rash itself is not infectious and symptomatic treatment only is required.

Other conditions

Henoch–Schonlein purpura (HSP)

■ Management group 2 – seek further advice from hospital

Like ITP, the importance of this condition is that whilst it presents with a purpuric rash, it is not an acute life-threatening condition. HSP classically affects children aged 3–8 years and is more common in boys. It often presents with a purpuric rash over the extensor surfaces of the buttocks and legs. Other common features are haematuria, proteinuria and joint pains. The condition is largely self-limiting although a small percentage of those affected may develop renal problems.

Eczema and psoriasis

■ Management group 3 – treat at home

Eczema and psoriasis are both chronic skin conditions that usually present in childhood and require treatment (albeit often intermittently) for life. This is usually initiated by the patient's GP, occasionally with input from a dermatologist. Whilst both conditions can frequently adversely affect a patient's quality of life, they rarely lead to serious complications that might present to an out-of-hours practitioner with two notable exceptions:

Infection

Either condition may become infected, usually as a result of the patient scratching at itchy lesions. This then requires the use of either a topical or oral antibiotic in addition to any ongoing treatment. Appropriate therapy should be initiated as described earlier (see cellulitis).

Pustular psoriasis

■ Management group 2 – seek further advice from hospital

Acute generalised pustular psoriasis is a rare but potentially life-threatening complication of psoriasis, usually requiring inpatient hospital treatment. As its name suggests, it presents in a patient with known psoriasis as widespread small pustules with areas of erythema, usually affecting the soles of the hands and/or feet. The pustules may coalesce to form large patches of pus. The condition may be precipitated by infection, pregnancy, or the withdrawal of steroid therapy. If suspected, consultation with a dermatologist or medical registrar on call is advised.

Other causes of isolated itching

■ Management group 3 – treat at home

Itching in isolation may be the presenting feature of a wide range of other clinical conditions (Table 12.7). All can be managed in the out-of-hours setting by the use of basic symptomatic measures and the patient should be advised to seek medical assessment thereafter.

TABLE 12.7 Clinical conditions associated with itch	
Cause	Comment
Senile itch	Occurs without an obvious cause in more than 50% of those aged >70 years and is thought to be linked to drying of the skin with age[1]
Cholestasis	Common symptom in jaundiced patients
Uraemia	Associated with chronic renal failure and affects approx 25% of those on haemodialysis. It may be limited to the site of a haemodialysis shunt
Solid tumours	Specific tumours are associated with localised itching: – scrotal itch with prostate cancer – itchy nostrils with brain tumours – vulval itch with cervical cancer – itch may also complicate chemotherapy
Blood disorders	Itch is frequently associated with disorders such as Hodgkin's lymphoma, leukaemia, myeloma and polycythaemia. It may also occur with iron deficiency anaemia
HIV	Itch is sometimes the first symptom of HIV-related disease

Basic symptomatic measures for the relief of itching

Itching in isolation is often associated with dry skin, so a moisturiser should be applied. The skin should be kept cool and the patient advised to avoid alcohol and spicy foods. Shower and bath water should be kept tepid to avoid further irritation.

No universally effective drug or cream exists for the relief of itching. Anti-histamine preparations in particular are only effective for itching caused by the release of histamine (e.g. insect bites). Creams containing a 1–2% mixture of menthol or phenol with aqueous cream can be applied topically several times a day for symptomatic relief of itching.[1]

Formulating a safe and effective management plan

Assess the patient's symptoms and signs to decide whether your patient needs emergency admission, semi-urgent admission or whether they can be safely treated at home:

1. Admit and treat *immediately* as an emergency (features of concern)
   Signs
   - Signs of airway obstruction
   - Respiratory rate <10 or >29
   - Oxygen saturation <92% on air
   - Pulse rate <50 or >120
   - Systolic BP <90
   - GCS <12
   Symptoms
   - Suspected rash of meningococcal septicaemia
   - Definite exposure to a trigger that has previously led to an anaphylactic reaction
   - Self-administration of epinephrine by a patient for a suspected anaphylactic reaction
   - A suspected anaphylactic reaction that has not fully developed
2. Admit as a semi-urgent case to hospital for further assessment and treatment
   Suspected cellulitis
   - Affecting the eyes or tissues around the eyes
   - Patient is 'unwell' (i.e. raised temperature, rigors, vomiting)
   - Patient unable to take oral antibiotics
   - No discernible clinical response to 24 hours of appropriate oral antibiotics
   - Other features of concern – e.g. gross pain or swelling, adverse social circumstances (lives alone, family unable to cope etc.)
3. Advisable to seek further advice from hospital
   - Purpuric rash but patient appears clinically well
   - Possible ITP or HSP
   - Possible pustular psoriasis
4. Can be treated at home, assuming no features of concern (as above)
   - Local allergic reactions
   - Urticaria/angioedema
   - Bacterial infections – mild cellulitis, impetigo, scarlet fever
   - Viral infections – chickenpox,[a,c] shingles,[a] measles,[a,b,c] rubella,[a,b,c] non-specific viral rashes [[a]Requires isolation to avoid spread (see text). [b]Notifiable disease in England and Wales (see above). [c]Notifiable disease in Scotland (see above)].

 PITFALL

Although this list aims to guide appropriate management, it is not foolproof. If in doubt, seek further medical advice

References

1 Twycross R, Greaves M W, Handwerker H et al 2003 Itch: scratching more than the surface. Q J Med 96:7–26

2 Woodward C M, Jessop E G, Wale M C 1995 Early management of meningococcal disease. Commun Dis Rep CDR Rev, 9:R135–137

3 McLean-Tooke A P, Bethune C A, Fay A C, Spickett G P 2003 Adrenaline in the treatment of anaphylaxis: what is the evidence?. BMJ 327:1332–1335

4 Brown A F, McKinnon D, Chu K 2001 Emergency department anaphylaxis: a review of 142 patients in a single year. J Allergy Clin Immunol 108:861–866

5 Kemp S F, Lockey R F, Wolf B L, Lieberman P 1995 Anaphylaxis. A review of 266 cases. Arch Intern Med 155:1749–1754

6 Noone M C, Osguthorpe J D 2003 Anaphylaxis. Otolaryngol Clin North Am 36:1009–1020

7 Simons F E R, Chad Z, Gold M 2002 Real-time reporting of anaphylaxis in infants, children and adolescents by physicians involved in the Canadian Pediatric Surveillance Program. J Allergy Clin Immunol 109:S181

8 Gupta R, Sheikh A, Strachan D, Anderson H R 2003 Increasing hospital admissions for systemic allergic disorders in England: analysis of national admissions data. BMJ 327:1142–1143

9 Simons F E, Gu X, Simons K J 2001 Epinephrine absorption in adults: intramuscular versus subcutaneous injection. J Allergy Clin Immunol 108:871–873

10 Tang A W 2003 A practical guide to anaphylaxis. Am Fam Phys 68: 1325–1332

11 Lieberman P 1990 The use of antihistamines in the prevention and treatment of anaphylaxis and anaphylactoid reactions. J Allergy Clin Immunol 86:684–686

12 Stark B J, Sullivan T J 1986 Biphasic and protracted anaphylaxis. J Allergy Clin Immunol 78:76–83

13 Ellis A K, Day J H 2003 Diagnosis and management of anaphylaxis. Can Med Assoc J 169:307–311

14 Hogan C 2002 Anaphylaxis. The GP perspective. Aust Fam Phys 31:807–809

15 British Association of Dermatologists Urticaria and Angioedema 2004 Available online: http://www.bad.org.uk/patients/disease (5 March 2007)

16 Grattan C, Powell S, Humphreys F 2001 Management and diagnostic guidelines for urticaria and angio-oedema. Br J Dermatol 144:708–714

17 Fay A, Abinun M 2002 Current management of hereditary angio-oedema (C′1 esterase inhibitor deficiency). J Clin Pathol 55:266–270

18 Health Protection Agency NOIDs Annual Totals 1994–2005 Available online: http://www.hpa.org.uk/infections/topics_az/noids/annualtab.htm (5 Mar 2007)

19 Surtees S J, Stockton M G, Gietzen T W 1991 Allergy to penicillin: fable or fact? BMJ 302:1051–1052

20 Begg N, Cartwright K A, Cohen J et al 1999 British Infection Society Working Party Consensus statement on diagnosis, investigation, treatment and prevention of acute bacterial meningitis in immunocompetent adults. J Infect 39:1–15

21 Baxter H, McGregor F 2001 Understanding and managing cellulitis. Nurs Stand 15(44):50–56

22 George A, Rubin G 2003 A systematic review and meta-analysis of treatments for impetigo. Br J Gen Pract 53:480–487

23 Hedrick J 2003 Acute bacterial skin infections in pediatric medicine: current issues in presentation and treatment. Paediatr Drugs 5(Suppl 1):35–46

24 Gnann J W Jr, Whitley R J 2002 Clinical practice. Herpes zoster. N Engl J Med 347:340–346

25 Duke T, Mgone C S 2003 Measles: not just another viral exanthema. Lancet 361:763–773

26 Wakefield A J, Murch S H, Anthony A et al 1998 Ileal-lymphoid-nodular hyperplasia, non-specific colitis, and pervasive developmental disorder in children. Lancet 351:637–641

27 Murch S 2003 Separating inflammation from speculation in autism. Lancet 362:1498–1499

Useful on-line resources

Allergy UK (UK) www.allergyuk.org (5 Mar 2007)

American Academy of Allergy, Asthma and Immunology www.aaaai.org (5 Mar 2007)

Anaphylaxis Canada www.anaphylaxis.org (5 Mar 2007)

British Association of Dermatologists (UK) www.bad.org.uk/about/ (5 Mar 2007)

Food Allergy and Anaphylaxis Network www.foodallergy.org (5 Mar 2007)

Health Protection Agency http://www.hpa.org.uk (5 Mar 2007)

Medic Alert Foundation (UK) www.medicalert.co.uk (5 Mar 2007)

Meningitis Research Foundation (UK) www.meningitis.org.uk (5 Mar 2007)

Platelet Disorder Support Association – Comprehensive web resource on ITP http://www.pdsa.org/ (5 Mar 2007)

Scottish Centre for Infection and Environmental Health www.show.scot.nhs.uk/scieh (5 Mar 2007)

UK-based Anaphylaxis campaign www.anaphylaxis.org.uk/ (5 Mar 2007)

World Allergy Organisation – List of worldwide allergy links http://www.worldallergy.org/links.shtml (5 Mar 2007)

Chris Fitzsimmons and Jim Wardrope

The assessment and care of musculoskeletal problems

Introduction

Musculoskeletal problems account for an estimated 3.5 million Emergency Department (ED) attendances each year. More patients will consult their general practitioner (GP) or treat the problem themselves. The majority of these conditions (sprains, bruises and aches) will be self-limiting, requiring clinical diagnosis, and straightforward treatment and advice.

However, there are diagnostic dilemmas facing the practitioner on the 'front line'. Even simple injuries often need hospital assessment, usually for X-rays. Some problems are rare but important to diagnose if life- or limb-threatening problems are to be avoided. The skill is to recognise those conditions where urgent referral and treatment are required. The aim of this chapter is to arm the practitioner with these skills (Box 13.1). Major trauma is not covered here.

BOX 13.1 **Chapter objectives**

- The recognition of life- or limb-threatening problems
- The identification of those patients requiring obvious hospital transfer
- The principles of a secondary survey relevant to musculoskeletal problems
- Differentiation between injury and non-injury presentations
- Differential diagnoses in non-injury musculoskeletal problems including pitfalls
- Follow-up arrangements
- An overview of the following will be included:
    - functional anatomy
    - forces causing injury and the injury spectrum
    - indications/regulations for X-rays
- Specific conditions to be covered:
    - back pain
    - neck pain
    - rib injury
    - degenerative disease/osteoarthritis
    - hot joints

The primary survey

Primary survey positive patients

Musculoskeletal injuries will rarely lead to a primary survey positive patient, except in major trauma. There are however immediately life-threatening problems that might mimic a musculoskeletal condition. These pose a trap for the unwary and are:

- leaking abdominal aortic aneurysm (AAA) presenting as back pain
- aortic dissection presenting as inter-scapular pain
- perforation/peritonitis presenting as shoulder tip pain
- acute myocardial infarction (MI) presenting as shoulder or arm pain.

A high index of suspicion and assessment of the ABCs can help identify these important conditions. A careful history will usually reveal no episode of trauma and a very acute onset of pain.

A leaking AAA presents acutely with abdominal and lower back pain with or without collapse and features of hypotension. The pain of an aortic dissection is described as tearing. Ischaemic chest pain is classically tight or band-like. Diaphragmatic irritation from a ruptured hollow viscus can cause shoulder pain, particularly on lying flat. Patients with these suspected conditions need urgent transport to a facility with the capabilities to fully manage these problems.

Immediate management will consist of essential interventions only. Administer oxygen, obtain intravenous access and give analgesia and possibly cautious fluid resuscitation en route. Do not delay transport to perform these procedures.

TIP

For further details on all these conditions see Chapters 3 and 9

Patients with a normal primary survey but obvious need for hospital attendance

Certain conditions pose a serious threat to life or limb and must not be missed when considering a 'wait-and-see' approach. The conditions listed in Box 13.2 are the 'red flag' conditions of the musculoskeletal system.

BOX 13.2 'Red flag' conditions requiring immediate hospital treatment

Trauma
- obvious fracture/dislocation
- open fracture
- severe pain not relieved by simple analgesia
- suspected compartment syndrome
- neurovascular compromise

Non-trauma
- referred pain from chest or abdomen
- ischaemia/vascular problems/suspected DVT
- septic arthritis/invasive soft tissue infections
- 'kids' problems such as slipped epiphysis
- neurological deficit, e.g. cauda equina syndrome

A *major joint dislocation* should be reduced as soon as possible, particularly if there is no distal circulation or sensation to the limb. Acutely ischaemic limbs need to have circulation restored within 4 hours to prevent irreversible muscle and nerve damage. Therefore make one gentle effort at relocation. Otherwise the limb needs to be splinted in its current position and urgent transfer arranged.

Compartment syndrome is caused by swelling in a myofascial compartment leading to a critically impaired circulation to the enclosed muscles in that compartment and possible distal ischaemia. There will usually be a good history of trauma. The hallmark of this condition is pain out of all proportion to the examination findings and exquisite pain on passive stretch of the muscles in the affected compartment. These patients require urgent transfer because surgical decompression is necessary as soon as possible, but certainly within 4 hours.

A septic joint is usually hot, swollen and very tender. All movements are restricted and it may be virtually impossible to move the joint due to pain. Typically the patient is systemically unwell and complains of the pain keeping them awake at night and being of a throbbing nature. These patients require urgent transfer to hospital because they need early surgery to remove the infection and preserve the joint.

Patients with objective *neurological deficit due to nerve root compression or due to other spinal pathology* should be referred immediately. Consider the diagnosis of a *cauda equina* syndrome. The lumbar and sacral nerve roots lie in the spinal canal below the level of L1/2. A central disc prolapse between the levels of L3 to S1 can compress these nerve roots causing retention of urine and weakness of the legs. The patient will present with lower back pain and neurological symptoms and signs. These include saddle area sensory loss and a reduced or absent anal tone on rectal examination. Depending on the level of the injury there will also be obvious neurological deficits in the motor assessment of the lower limbs.

The minimum necessary interventions should be carried out on these patients but could include administration of oxygen or entonox, splinting, dressing open wounds, IV analgesia and controlled traction or reduction of neurovascularly compromised extremities. These procedures should not delay transfer arrangements.

> ### TIP
>
> For further information on the treatment of compartment syndrome and crush syndrome see the ATLS manual[1] and Wardrope.[2] For dislocations, septic joints and neurovascular compromise see Wardrope,[2] Apley,[3] and McRae[4]

Secondary survey patients

Assessment of the stable patient

The assessment is carried out according to the recognised system (SOAPC) outlined in Chapter 2. The first step is to decide if the problem is due to *trauma* or one of the many causes of *non-traumatic limb or spinal pain*. The spectrum of diagnoses is very different in these two groups.

TIP

The first step in the assessment of musculoskeletal symptoms is to decide if the problem is due to an episode of trauma or a non-traumatic problem

Trauma vs no history of trauma

Patients who present with no history of trauma should alert the clinician to the possibility of missing **R**eferred pain, **I**schaemic syndromes, **S**epsis and **K**ids problems such as epiphyseal abnormalities. Remember the mnemonic **RISK**. These are the conditions commonly overlooked and can indicate limb- or even life-threatening problems such as cardiac pain, a slipped upper femoral epiphysis or a septic joint.

Subjective information gathering – the history

Definite trauma

Acute trauma is caused by a single, clear event. This can lead to a wide spectrum of injury from minor self-limiting sprains to fractures and/or dislocations of joints. The features of a fracture are pain, swelling, loss of function and bony tenderness. Dislocations are usually more obvious with similar features to fractures plus an abnormal joint morphology with deformity. In the absence of these features then a soft tissue injury is more likely but consider damage to other structures such as ligaments, tendons, nerves and vessels (Box 13.3).

BOX 13.3 The elements of history taking in acute trauma

- Mechanism of injury
- Symptoms and progress of symptoms over time
- Previous episodes of injury
- Past medical history/drugs/allergy
- Level of activity in job or sport

Mechanism of injury

A clear history of the mechanism of injury is essential to accurate diagnosis in trauma. Elicit the magnitude and direction of the forces causing the injury. Simple errors are made by a failure to follow this advice. For example, if the only history obtained was 'hurt neck in road traffic accident' the clinician might jump to the conclusion the injury was likely to be a simple neck sprain. However, consider how different your actions might be if a full history were to be obtained such as 'hurt neck in road traffic accident, was unrestrained front seat passenger in car which overturned at speed' (Fig. 13.1).

Symptoms and progress

Pain, swelling and loss of function are the main symptoms following injury. Ask if these symptoms have progressed since the incident. A sudden and complete loss of function at time of impact increases the risk

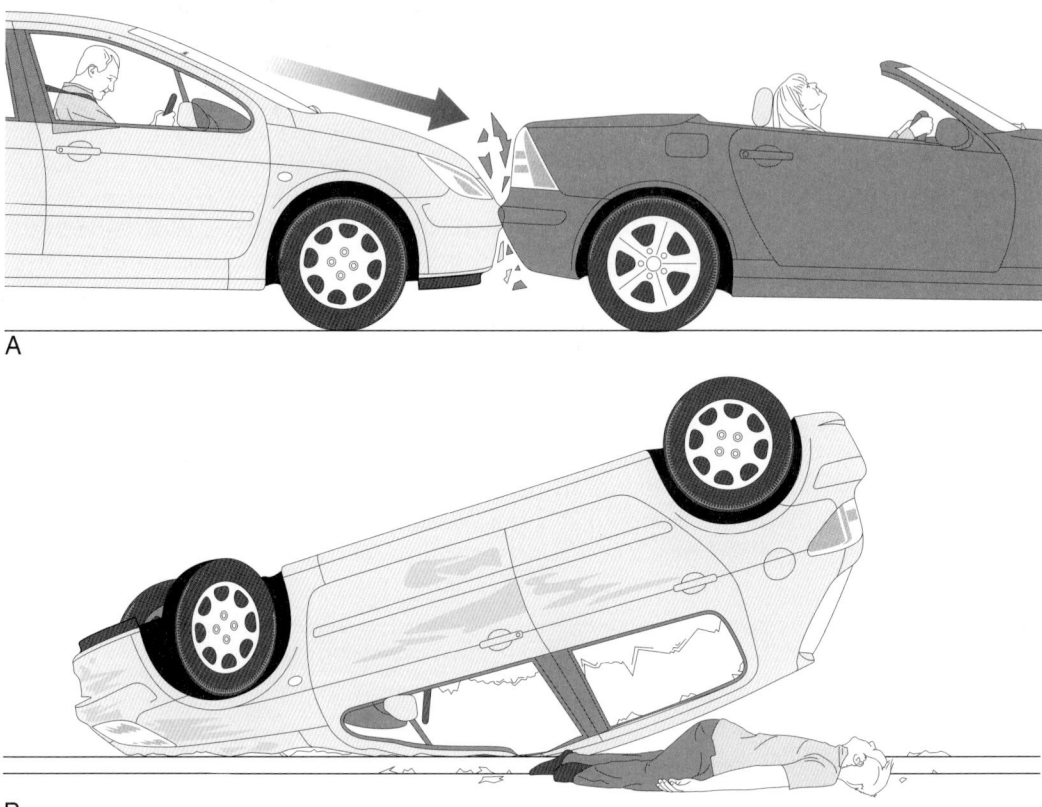

A

B

Fig. 13.1   A history of 'hurt neck in road traffic accident' can mean anything from the injury being sustained in a minor rear end shunt to a major high speed and high risk impact. Always try to gain a clear mental picture of the mechanics of the injury.

for a more severe injury. Ask about associated symptoms such as paraesthesia and trauma elsewhere.

Past history and previous injuries

Ask the patient if they have any other significant medical conditions or are taking any medication. Most injuries are acute, but some are an acute episode complicating a chronic problem. The investigation and treatment of an 'acute on chronic' injury may be slightly different.

Level of activity

Patient expectations are an important consideration in the management of musculoskeletal injuries. A professional athlete will demand as near 100% function as is possible post-injury but most patients will manage very well with minor ligament instability as long as they have good protective neuromuscular function. Nevertheless it is important to consider occupation, hobbies and handedness so that expectations and needs can be identified.

No definite trauma

Patients who present with a limb or spinal pain but with no history of trauma can present diagnostic problems. In the majority of patients the illness will be minor and self-limiting or of a chronic nature not needing urgent treatment or investigation. However a minority of patients with these 'minor' symptoms may be suffering from life- or limb-threatening pathology. The mnemonic 'RISK' highlights the categories of serious diagnoses that may require exclusion (Box 13.4). *Always* consider the RISK diagnoses – failure to do so *will* lead to them being missed.

BOX 13.4 'RISK' diagnoses in non-traumatic limb and spinal pain

- R   Referred pain from chest/abdomen/spine*
- I   Ischaemia/vascular problems/DVT
- S   Sepsis
- K   Kids problems such as an epiphyseal injury

*Examples include shoulder pain due to irritation of the diaphragm or knee pain due to hip pathology.

History in non-traumatic limb and spinal pain

TIP

Severe pain at night – consider severe pathology

The most common symptom is pain. OPQRST is a good mnemonic to help remember the questions that should be asked about pain (see below). Many serious pathologies cause severe pain with few findings on examination. Pain at night that keeps the patient awake is of special significance. It usually indicates a severe inflammatory process and should always be taken seriously.

The 'OPQRST' of pain

See Box 13.5.

BOX 13.5 'OPQRST' history taking of the symptom of pain

- O – onset
- P – provoking and palliative factors
- Q – quality
- R – referred pain
- S – systemic symptoms/associate symptoms
- T – timing

O – Onset

A very sudden onset of pain is often associated with a vascular problem such as occlusion or referred pain from cardiac ischaemia or a leaking aortic aneurysm. Sudden pain waking the patient at night is a worrying symptom. Some mechanical problems do cause a sudden onset of pain in the absence of definite trauma, examples include an acute intervertebral disc prolapse or a loose body in a joint. Many other causes of limb pain will cause a gradual onset or intermittent symptoms.

P – Provoking or palliative factors

Ask if the patient has participated in any unusual activity in the period leading up to the onset of symptoms, or has recently significantly increased the level of an activity (e.g. doubling their running distance) which would be unusual for that patient. Note other aggravating or relieving factors.

Q – Quality of pain

Is the pain throbbing in nature, toothache-like, or sharp and associated with certain movements? How severe is the pain?

R – Radiation and site

Ask if the pain radiates either proximally or distally in the limb. This may be an indication that the problem lies more centrally. Common examples are:

- arm pain radiating from the neck or heart
- shoulder pain from irritation of the diaphragm
- knee pain from the hip and leg pain from the lumbar spine.

S – Systemic symptoms/associated symptoms/ previous history

Does the patient have markers of a systemic illness such as fever, chills, loss of appetite or weight loss?

Joint problems are sometimes associated with systemic illnesses. Ask if there are any other symptoms such as back problems (ankylosing spondylitis), eye problems, inflammatory bowel symptoms, genitourinary symptoms, recent illnesses, and respiratory tract infection. Some types of acute arthritis are part of complex syndromes, e.g. Reiter's syndrome.

Note previous medical history, especially if there have been similar problems in the past. Exclude problems with other joints or a history of arthritis. Exclude many of the more common diseases such as diabetes. Does the patient take warfarin or have any coagulopathy?

T – Timing

Does the pain keep the patient awake at night? Is it worse first thing in the morning or after exercise?

Objective information gathering – the examination

Develop a systematic method of musculoskeletal examination:

- joint above
- look
- feel
- move
- function
- nerves and vessels.

TIP

See Chapter 2 on examination, including the musculoskeletal system. See also Wardrope,[2] Cyriax[5] and McRae[6] for a fuller examination description of anatomical regions

Have the patient in a relaxed position. Start by examining the joint proximal to the injury (or spine if indicated). Follow standard orthopaedic practice, using the 'look, feel, move, function' system. Finish by checking the circulation to the limbs and test neural function distal to the injury.

Where there is no history of trauma, follow the same system but check vital signs and look for other clinical signs as summarised in Box 13.6.

BOX 13.6 Clinical signs to look for when there is no history of trauma

- Vital signs – particularly temperature and pulse rate
- Stigmata of systemic disease or of systemic arthritis
- Skin rashes
- Proximal joints
- Neurovascular examination
- Spine
- (Chest and abdomen if indicated)

Objective information – tests

X-Rays – indications

If a fracture or dislocation is suspected then the patient needs referral to hospital. Many will need immediate referral, but if there is no deformity, no neurovascular compromise and the injured limb can be effectively immobilised (including non weight bearing for the lower limb) the patient might be referred for X-ray at a more convenient time. Outpatient referral to the radiology department of the local hospital allows non-urgent X-rays to be performed. Many departments have a system of 'hot reporting' so that X-rays are reviewed immediately. If abnormalities are seen the patient is referred to the appropriate hospital team. If X-rays are normal the patient may return to their GP for further treatment.

Use local guidelines and policy to decide when an X-ray is indicated. The definite fractures are easy to diagnose but unfortunately many fractures are undisplaced and it is difficult to confidently exclude a fracture without an X-ray. Many experienced clinicians would advise 'X-ray when

Fig. 13.2 Ottawa ankle rules.

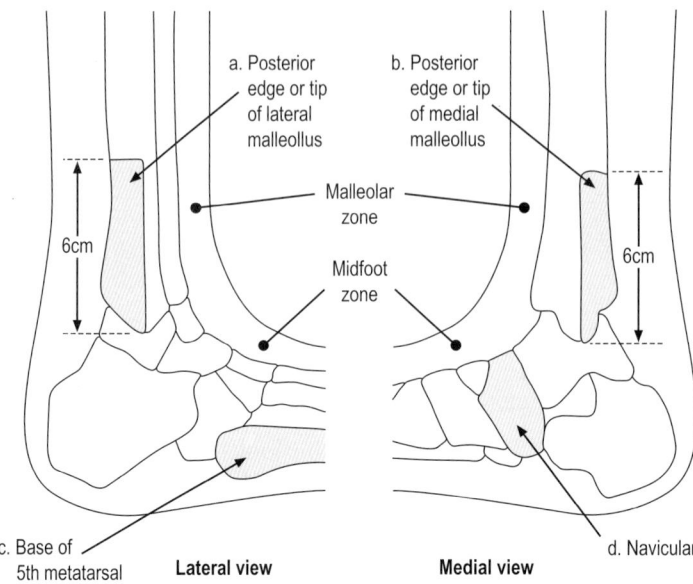

a. Posterior edge or tip of lateral malleollus

b. Posterior edge or tip of medial malleollus

Malleolar zone

Midfoot zone

6cm

6cm

c. Base of 5th metatarsal

Lateral view

d. Navicular

Medial view

in doubt'. Other indications include suspected foreign body within a wound, e.g. glass or metal. For further information see the Royal College of Radiologists guidance on www.rcr.ac.uk and 'Making the best use of a Department of Clinical Radiology'.[7]

There are other excellent reference sources available for the need to X-ray certain anatomical areas such as the ankle. Probably the best known are the Ottawa ankle rules[8] used to help decision making in the assessment of acute ankle injuries that may either be sprained (the majority) or fractured (Fig. 13.2).

Other decision rules exist for similar use in acute knee[9] and neck[10] injuries.

Be aware that many of these decision tools have limited applicability to groups such as the elderly, whose bones may fracture more easily, and very young children, where epiphyseal injuries may be more common. The Ottawa ankle rules have however been validated in children down to the age of 6 years.

In January 2000 the Ionising Radiation (Medical Exposures) Regulations came into force to protect patients undergoing exposure to X-rays. Any clinician ordering X-rays independently needs to be accredited and attend training on this subject. For further information on IRMER legislation see the Department of Health website (www.dh.gov.uk/assetRoot/04/05/78/38/04057838.pdf).

Investigations – no definite trauma

Many patients will not require any immediate investigation and may be referred to their GP for further assessment. However if you suspect any of the RISK diagnoses, investigations such as blood tests, examination of joint fluid, ultrasound, bone scans and CT or MRI scanning may be required. In addition, X-rays of the area may be required – but note that many serious conditions may have an initially normal X-ray.

Analysis and differential diagnosis

Trauma

A 'sprain' is a tear in a ligament and the term covers a huge spectrum of injury, from the minor partial tear of a part of a ligament to a permanently disabling injury. A careful history and examination allows the definition of the severity and builds an accurate picture of the likely damage caused:

- grade 1 sprain is where a few fibres of part of the ligament are torn
- grade 2 sprain is complete rupture of part of the ligament complex, e.g. rupture of the anterior talo-fibular ligament of the ankle lateral ligament complex
- grade 3 sprain is complete disruption of the ligament complex with associated instability.

Great difficulty arises in the grading of ligament injury. Grade 3 injuries are usually clinically obvious, with much more bruising and swelling. Instability is the main concern mandating aggressive treatment, splintage, referral, repair and/or physiotherapy. A repeat examination after 5 days may be needed to establish the true extent of some injuries. Use a 'wait-and-see' policy as long as you have excluded a potentially serious injury.

Muscle tears or strains are common and usually self-limiting. Some muscles and tendons can rupture completely; the most common closed ligament injury is rupture of the Achilles tendon. This diagnosis may be missed if not specifically tested.

Fractures are often easy to diagnose but are difficult to exclude. Pitfalls include the scaphoid fracture in adults, hip fractures in the elderly and spinal fractures. Osteogenesis imperfecta (brittle bone disease) should lead to a very high index of suspicion for fracture even with minimal trauma.

No definite trauma

Common diagnoses are osteoarthritis (OA) and degenerative disease. Ask about previous symptoms (these are discussed below).

- Consider referred pain, ischaemia, sepsis and kids (RISK) as causes of pain when no other cause seems apparent. Limb pain could be due to a septic joint, a critical ischaemia or referred from spine, abdomen or chest.

- Causes of a 'hot joint' include gout, pseudogout, infection, acute arthritis and haematological conditions – see below.
- Beware children. The slipped upper femoral epiphysis is the classic pitfall where minimal or no trauma is involved yet a significant pathology occurs that needs to be appreciated as early as possible for corrective treatment to commence.

Plan

Many musculoskeletal problems can be treated by simple advice, analgesia and review by the patient's GP.

Most minor musculoskeletal injuries can be treated by advising the patient to rest the injured area for the first 24–48 hours, to take regular analgesia, to elevate the injured part if possible. Sometimes the application of cold compresses may reduce swelling. However the most important advice is to try to retain mobility by gentle exercise and a gradual return to full function. Tell the patient to seek further review if the pain gets worse or does not start to improve in 3–5 days. It may take weeks for symptoms to subside fully.

Communication

The successful management of most minor musculoskeletal injuries depends on the patient understanding the importance of phased rehabilitation as described above. Equally they should be encouraged to seek early review by their GP if the symptoms are worsening.

Specific problems

Back pain

One very common problem is acute *mechanical back pain*, this usually occurs in young fit people. The pain usually starts suddenly and is often severe. However, if there are no 'red flag' symptoms (Box 13.7), advice is given to try to stay mobile and good analgesia prescribed. Cases with unusual or continuing severe symptoms should be reviewed early by their GP.

Pain radiating down the back of the leg to below the knee may indicate sciatic nerve irritation. A careful neurological examination is needed. Refer for early review by the GP.[11] If there is pain down both legs or any disturbance of motor power, bladder or bowel function, then refer to hospital immediately.

There are many other causes of back pain. Severe pain, an insidious onset, systemic symptoms and onset with no history of trauma should all lead to consideration of other causes such as referred pain, infection, tumour and spinal cord compression. An acute onset with collapse, sweatiness and pallor should alert you to the possibility of a leaking AAA. Always take seriously any altered sensory or motor findings in the lower limbs. The examination of the lower back is not complete without a full neurovascular assessment, abdominal examination and an examination of the saddle area for sensation. (Rectal examination to assess tone is usually advised but may be difficult in the community setting.)

Consider referral if the cause is not completely clear for further assessment and possible X-ray, FBC, ESR, CRP and even CT or MRI scanning in certain cases. Remember to complete a full systems examination first, documenting important findings such as the pulse rate and temperature.

Box 13.7 shows 'red flags' that might indicate serious spinal pathology in back pain (adapted from the Report of Clinical Standards Advisory Group on Back Pain[11]).

BOX 13.7 'Red flags' that might indicate serious spinal pathology

History
- age <20 or >50 at onset
- Trauma (fall from height/RTA)
- Thoracic pain
- Constant, progressive pain
- Weight loss

PMH
- Carcinoma
- Steroid use
- Drug abuse/HIV

Examination
- Systemically unwell
- Persisting severe restriction of lumbar flexion
- Widespread neurology
- Structural deformity (scoliosis/step)

Neck pain

Causes include whiplash injury, torticollis, referred pain, degenerative disease and infection. As with back pain, a good history of trauma will allow an assessment of the neck for injury such as fracture dislocation.

BOX 13.8 'Clearing the C-spine' after trauma

Patients fulfilling these criteria will have a very low incidence of unstable spinal injury and may not need an X-ray:

- Younger than 65
- Alert and orientated (GCS = 15)
- No 'dangerous mechanism of injury':
    - fall from a height above 1 metre, fall from 5 or more stairs
    - axial load to the head such as diving or contact sports
    - RTA at high speed, rollover of vehicle or ejection of patient
    - RTA involving bicycle or recreational vehicle
    - rear-end shunt by a bus, vehicle at high speed or where car has been shunted into oncoming traffic
    - in young children have a lower index of suspicion in falls
- No midline spinal tenderness
- No neurological symptoms or signs
- Patient can rotate neck 45 degrees to left and right
- Absence of a distracting injury (e.g. long bone fracture)

Guidance on how to 'clear the C-spine' after trauma has been issued by NICE[12] and Stiell[10] and is summarised by Wardrope[13] (Box 13.8).

Whiplash is very common after minor road traffic accidents. Pain comes on after a period of time, usually several hours to days. It is classically aching and worse on one side than the other. Sometimes it is entirely unilateral but is more usually bilateral. Assess for range of movement and neurovascular problems. Treatment is by gentle mobilisation, NSAIDs, advice and an explanation that symptoms often worsen before they begin to improve and will commonly take weeks to months to settle fully.

Torticollis is an acute neck pain with associated muscle spasm. It occurs most commonly in young fit patients who often wake up with the pain, stiffness and greatly decreased range of movement. Muscle spasm is seen and felt in the corresponding neck muscles unilaterally. There is no history of trauma or of infection. Treat with NSAIDs and gentle mobilisation of the neck.

Infection and *tumour* are rare. Consider them in the same manner as such conditions anywhere else in the body and have a low threshold for referral to hospital if suspected from the history or unusual physical findings such as fever, systemic symptoms or unexplained tachycardia.

Degenerative disease/osteoarthritis

These chronic progressive conditions can affect any region of the body, but most commonly are encountered in the hip, knee and cervical and lumbar spine. They may present as a new problem, an acute flare up of the chronic condition after relatively minor trauma, or as a more significant injury or infection superimposed on coincidental findings of degenerative disease.

Ask about trauma stiffness or problems with other major joints. Check other joints for swelling, stiffness and crepitus on movement. An arthritic joint is more likely to become inflamed after trauma and symptoms and signs may be harder to interpret than in the non-arthritic joint.

The classic example of this is the elderly patient who has fallen and has hip pain. The diagnosis to exclude is a fractured neck of femur. Contrary to popular belief, patients can walk on such injuries, especially if the fracture is impacted and stable. If not X-raying, consider early review to ensure good mobility and settling symptoms.

Rib injuries

These injuries are common and often present after relatively minor trauma. Acute rib injuries are very painful and present with pain that is often apparently out of proportion to the initial injury. Presentation is often several days after the injury when the pain may be worse than at the time of injury. Fracture is not as common as bruising and soft tissue injury to the chest wall, but the features can be almost identical. 'Spring' the chest wall in a lateral and antero-posterior (AP) direction to assess for pain and crepitus. This is also felt when the patient takes a deep breath with the examining hand held firmly over the injured area. Listen for areas of reduced air entry or added sounds suggesting underlying pneumothorax, contusion or early infection. Examine the abdomen in cases of lower rib injury. Check pulse, temperature, respiratory rate and oxygen saturation (SaO_2) if available.

Rib X-rays are not routinely indicated but arrange a chest X-ray if the patient is short of breath at rest or on minimal exercise, if there is suspicion of a pneumothorax, there is clinical suspicion that multiple ribs are fractured, there is a flail segment present or infection has complicated the injury. For uncomplicated rib injury the management includes advice on breathing exercises and good analgesia.

Patients may need referral, particularly the elderly or those with pre-existing lung disease and a poor respiratory reserve. They may need stronger analgesia and supplemental oxygen.

The acutely hot/swollen/painful joint

Pain, swelling and redness in the region of a joint may be due to a condition within the joint (acute arthritis) or in the tissues around the joint (periarthritis).

The commonest problems causing an acutely swollen, hot joint are the crystal arthropathies of *gout* and *pseudogout* and acute inflammatory conditions such as *rheumatoid arthritis*. *Sepsis* is relatively rare but is a diagnosis not to be missed. Acute haemarthrosis is uncommon without a history of trauma, coagulopathy or anticoagulant treatment.

Bursitis is a common condition that presents with pain, swelling and redness *around* joints. However there is no swelling in the joint itself and a reasonable range of joint movement is retained. Very common examples are olecranon bursitis behind the elbow and pre- and infra-patellar bursitis at the knee. Sometimes degenerative changes in tendons lead to calcium pyrophosphate crystals developing in the tendon. This can give a clinical picture of a red, hot, swollen area over a joint.

Degenerative disease such as *osteoarthritis* often causes joint swelling but the joint is not usually hot and red (Box 13.9).

Gout occurs when crystals of uric acid from the blood precipitate in a joint, causing an intense and acute inflammation of the joint. *Pseudogout* is a very similar condition caused by deposition of calcium pyrophosphate crystals. Both can present as a red, hot, painful and swollen joint. The skin overlying a gouty joint is often tight, red and shiny. The pain has a classic deep, gnawing character and the patient often has suffered previous attacks. It commonly affects the first metatarsophalangeal joint of the foot but also affects the ankle and less commonly the knee. Pseudogout tends to affect the wrist, where calcification is sometimes seen in the triangular ligament on X-ray; and the knee, where calcification may be apparent in the meniscal cartilage.

Where the patient has a clear history of previous gout, treatment is with non-steroidal anti-inflammatory drugs (NSAIDs). In a typical case of gout or pseudogout where the patient is well, has no systemic symptoms of infection and is apyrexial, give a short course of NSAIDs and arrange next day review by the GP.

The diagnoses not to miss are *osteomyelitis* and *septic arthritis*. Septic arthritis can arise de novo or from spread from an area of osteomyelitis into the joint. They both present in a similar way. There is either no history of trauma or a history of insignificant trauma for the degree of pain. There may be a history of joint penetration, either in an accident

---

BOX 13.9 Causes of an acute hot swelling in or around a joint

Acute arthritis
- Gout
- Pseudogout
- Sero-positive arthritis (e.g. rheumatoid)
- Sero-negative arthritis (e.g. Reiter's syndrome)
- Sepsis
- Haemarthrosis

Peri-arthritis
- Bursitis
- CPPDD (calcium pyrophosphate deposition disease)

or caused by a medical intervention. The patient cannot move the joint at all and strongly resists any passive movements. Early in the course of these illnesses, all these classical findings may not be present. Consider sepsis a possibility in any acute joint problem and arrange for early review. If in doubt refer for a further opinion to the patient's GP, rheumatology or A&E.

Haemophilia and *sickle cell disease* are both haematological disorders that can result in acute joint pain from either bleeding into the joint or ischaemia and infarction of tissues around the area. Refer urgently if the patient has a history of these conditions.

References

1 American College of Surgeons Committee on Trauma 1997 ATLS manual, 6th edn. American College of Surgeons, Chicago
2 Wardrope J, English B 1998 Musculoskeletal problems in emergency medicine, 1st edn. Oxford University Press, Oxford
3 Apley A G, Solomon L 1995 Apley's system of orthopaedics and fractures, 7th edn. Butterworth-Heinemann, Oxford
4 McRae R 1994 Practical fracture management, 3rd edn. Churchill Livingstone, Edinburgh
5 Cyriax J H, Cyriax P J 1993 Cyriax's illustrated manual of orthopaedic medicine, 2nd edn. Butterworth-Heinemann, Oxford
6 McRae R 1997 Clinical orthopaedic examination. Churchill Livingstone, Edinburgh
7 Royal College of Radiologists 2003 Making the best use of a department of clinical radiology. Guidelines for doctors, 5th edn. RCR, London
8 Stiell I G, Greenberg G H, McKnight R D, Nair R C, McDowell I, Worthington J R 1992 A study to develop clinical decision rules for the use of radiography in acute ankle injuries. Ann Emerg Med 21:384–390
9 Stiell I G, Greenberg G H, Wells G A et al 1996 Prospective validation of a decision rule for the use of radiography in acute knee injuries. JAMA 275(8):611–615
10 Stiell I G, Wells G A, Vandemheen K L et al 2001 The Canadian C-spine rule for radiography in alert and stable trauma patients. JAMA 286(15):1841–1848
11 Clinical Standards Advisory Group 1994 Report of the Clinical Standards Advisory Group on Back Pain. HMSO, London
12 National Institute for Health and Clinical Excellence 2003 Head injury: triage, assessment, investigation and early management of head injury in infants, children and adults. Clinical Practice Algorithm No. 4. NICE, London
13 Wardrope J, Ravichandran G, Locker T 2004 Risk assessment for spinal injury after trauma. BMJ 328:721–723

Web references

Emedicine– www.emedicine.com (5 Mar 2007)
Royal College of Radiologists– www.rcr.ac.uk (5 Mar 2007)
Department of Health– www.dh.gov.uk (5 Mar 2007)

Jim Wardrope and Peter Driscoll

Overdose and self harm

Primary survey positive patient

TIP

Request immediate back up when dealing with primary survey positive patients

The objectives of this chapter are listed in Box 14.1. Poisoning and self-inflicted trauma are two of the commonest causes of death and life-threatening emergencies in patients less than 40 years of age. These will present as primary positive patients for the reasons listed in Box 14.2. However be aware that these can be compounded by major trauma as part of the suicide attempt (e.g. falls, hanging and shootings). Recognition and management of these associated injuries are described elsewhere.

BOX 14.1 Chapter objectives

■ The management of immediately life-threatening problems
■ The secondary survey including issues of consent
■ Signs and symptoms associated with overdoses of particular drugs

---

BOX 14.2 Life threatening problems in overdose

■ *Airway*
  ■ unconscious patient, airway obstruction
  ■ vomit in airway
  ■ asphyxia (hanging)
  ■ penetrating trauma to neck
■ *Breathing*
  ■ respiratory depression (opiates)
  ■ carbon monoxide poisoning
  ■ penetrating trauma to chest
  ■ aspiration
■ *Circulation*
  ■ drug-induced hypotension
  ■ drug-induced cardiac arrhythmia
  ■ blood loss (wrists/neck injury)
  ■ hyperpyrexia
■ *Disability*
  ■ unconscious patient – hypoglycaemia, sedative drugs, fits
  ■ lack of capacity to consent to treatment and threatening suicide
■ *Environmental*
  ■ hypothermia

Management

As you are assessing the ABCs, take a history or look for clues that might indicate the cause. Often it is obvious but in the unconscious patient it may not be.

The airway

The care of the airway is discussed in Chapter 2. Usually good basic techniques, such as airway opening procedures and patient positioning will be sufficient. Do the least to ensure a clear airway as in some types of drug overdose over aggressive intervention might induce vomiting or extreme bradycardia.

Breathing

Opiate overdose is the commonest cause of drug-induced hypoventilation. The initial management is to open the airway and ventilate using bag/valve mask techniques. Naloxone is a very effective antidote but can wear off before the opiate has been removed from the body. Consequently if the patient wakes up and then refuses to go to hospital, there is a risk that respiratory depression may re-occur once the naloxone is metabolised. As this has led to patients dying JRCALC recommends the titration of the naloxone to keep the patient in a 'groggy state'. In such circumstances we recommend that naloxone is given slowly to bring the respiratory rate above 10 breaths per minute.

Carbon monoxide poisoning due to attempted suicide is usually diagnosed by the circumstances (e.g. a pipe from the car exhaust threaded through the vehicle's side window). Accidental carbon monoxide poisoning can be very difficult to diagnose. Important clues are finding one or more people from the same enclosed space presenting with neurological signs such as headache, confusion and unconsciousness. In these circumstances have the area checked for a carbon monoxide source such as a room or water heater with poor ventilation. These patients must be removed from the poisonous environment, provided with high flow oxygen as part of basic ABC care and transported to hospital.

Circulation

Life-threatening haemorrhage occasionally occurs in those who have self harmed by cutting a major blood vessel. Management entails stemming the source of the bleeding by direct pressure and rapidly transporting the patient to hospital. During the journey IV access can be obtained but do not infuse large amounts of fluid as this is likely to increase the blood loss. Instead give enough fluid to maintain a radial pulse.

Many drugs can cause hypotension; Box 14.3 lists the commonest. The initial management is to obtain IV access, to give fluids and arrange transport to hospital. Simple measures such as raising the legs are also effective. The commonest drugs causing arrhythmia are listed in Box 14.4.

If the arrhythmia is immediately life-threatening, treat along Advanced Life Support guidelines. In most circumstances however the only interventions which are required are IV access, monitoring and transport to hospital. There are specific treatments for beta-blocker and antidepressant overdose but it will depend on local policy if these are implemented at scene.

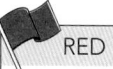

RED FLAG

Any patient given naloxone should be taken to hospital. If they refuse you must make all attempts to persuade them to go. Failing this, arrange for someone to observe them for 6 hours and make arrangements for a follow-up call within 2–3 hours

---

BOX 14.3 **Drugs causing hypotension**

- Alcohol
- Tricyclic antidepressant drugs
- Opiates
- Beta-blockers
- Calcium antagonists
- Iron

> **BOX 14.4 Drugs causing arrhythmia**
>
> - *Bradycardia*
>   - beta-blockers
> - *Tachycardia*
>   - antidepressants
>   - cocaine
>   - amphetamines
>   - ecstasy
> - *SVT/VT*
>   - antidepressants

Hyperpyrexia is a specific complication of sympathomimetic drugs such as ecstasy and SSRIs. The management is again to obtain IV access, monitor and immediate transfer to hospital.

Disability

If the patient is unconscious, call for immediate back up. Check and manage the airway, breathing and circulation. Always check the blood sugar level.

Alcohol, opiates, antidepressant drugs and benzodiazepines are the commonest drugs to cause a reduced conscious level. Antidepressant drugs can, in addition, cause bizarre behaviour or an acute confusional state.

Fitting due to poisoning indicates severe intoxication but the management remains the same (see Chapter 10). Clear the airway, position the patient, administer oxygen, gain IV access (check the blood glucose) and if needed, give diazepam or lorazepam.

Refusal of treatment by a patient who is threatening suicide is one of the most difficult situations to manage. The reason may be the patient's lack of capacity to make an informed decision. You will need help. Family, friends or carers are often the most effective in negotiating with the patient and gaining agreement to take the patient to hospital. Alternatively the patient may have regular contact with mental health services or their general practitioner who could be called for advice. The majority of cases will be resolved by negotiation. However there will be some extreme cases where there is an obvious, immediate and real threat to life and when the patient is refusing treatment. If you think the patient lacks capacity to make a reasoned decision then there is a conflict between your responsibility to act in the best interests of the patient and the patient's rights. There is no 'right' answer to such cases as all are different. You must involve other professionals. In extreme circumstances you may have to treat the patient against their wishes, this may require the police. See Chapter 15 for a full discussion on consent, capacity and treatment against the patient's wishes.

Environment

If the patient has been immobile and unconscious for some time, they may be hypothermic. Pressure sores, aspiration pneumonia and renal failure are other complications. In addition to basic resuscitation care, treat by gradual re-warming, minimal intervention and transport to hospital.

Activated charcoal

This consists of very small particles of charcoal which bind to the drug in the gastrointestinal tract. Its aim is therefore to prevent the toxins absorption into the circulation. It can be used for most poisons but there are some notable exceptions (Box 14.5).

BOX 14.5 Activated charcoal

Activated charcoal does not work for:
- metals (Fe, lithium, Hg)
- acid and alkali
- alcohols (ethanol, ethylene glycol, methanol)
- organic solvents

As activated charcoal comes in a powder form, water is added so it can be drunk by the patient. As most people find it unpalatable it is often pre-mixed with flavoured drinks. The patient also needs to be conscious with an intact airway as aspiration of activated charcoal can lead to significant respiratory complications.

Close observation is required if the airway is at slightest risk and activated charcoal has been administered.

There is no good evidence that activated charcoal has any effect on the outcome of overdose. However its use is recommended by NICE in patients who have taken a life-threatening overdose within one hour of them being assessed. Its use by primary care personnel will therefore depend on local circumstances and protocols.

Conditions that will require transport to hospital

At present most patients with self harm are taken to hospital where they can receive treatment for both the physical and psychological problems. The former invariably consists of investigations and a period of observation.

This regimen may change in the future as mental health services are resourced to respond to urgent needs in the community. However transfer to hospital will remain the best way to access support services where these services are not fully operational.

Secondary survey

Subjective information

There are currently few specific tests routinely available in the community that will assist in diagnosing and managing overdoses. History taking and examination are therefore very important (Box 14.6). The identity of any drugs taken, the amount taken and the time of the overdose are the critical parts of the medical history. Check if other drugs or alcohol have been taken. Record any symptoms such as drowsiness, nausea, vomiting. Note the past medical history and current medications. Refer to the British National Formulary or Toxbase for symptoms associated with a specific drug.

Carry out a general screening examination and any specific examination as suggested by patient symptoms or BNF/Toxbase advice. Very often the examination will be normal. Record the vital signs, the mental state assessment and suicide risk (see Chapter 15). The psychological assessment is as important as the physical one. Chapter 15 outlines the assessment of suicide risk and psychiatric examination. The social history is also very important – especially the availability of immediate social support.

BOX 14.6 Key information in the toxin history

- What taken?
- When?
- What else?
- How much?
- Why?

Assessment

The diagnosis of the physical problem and risk is usually straight forward. The assessment of the psychological state and suicide risk is much less certain.

Each year people with depression account for two-thirds of all deaths from suicide nationally. Risk assessment tools and rating scales can be very helpful, e.g. the Suicide and Self-Harm Risk Assessment Scale, this can most easily be remembered using the SADPERSONS acronym (Box 14.7).

Plan

Most patients with significant self harm will need to go to hospital. Occasionally if the overdose has been very minor, the suicidal risk is judged to be low and there is good social back up, a case might be made for treating the patient at home with referral to primary care or for appropriate psychological support.

BOX 14.7 **SADPERSONS risk stratification**

Score 3 or less, low risk; 3–6 medium risk, more than 6 high risk (this is a guide only and should not be used to replace clinical judgement)

- Sex male   1
- Age <19 or >45   1
- Depression/hopelessness   2
- Previous attempts   1
- Excessive alcohol/drugs   1
- Rational thinking (loss of)   2
- Separated widowed divorced   1
- Organised or serious attempt   1
- No social support   1
- Stated future intent   2

Specific poisons

Full details of the effects of each drug can be found in standard texts or in Toxbase. This section highlights the problems associated with each class of drug and the pitfalls.

Aspirin overdose

This commonly available drug can produce a range of symptoms that approximate to its plasma level 4 hours after ingestion (Table 14.1).

Management

At scene there is no specific treatment for an aspirin overdose. Provide basic ABC care, measure the BM (as it can be low) and transport the patient to hospital. Upon arrival therapy is directed at minimising further GI absorption, gastric irritation and preventing organ failure.

Beta blockers

Beta blocker overdose causes around 20 deaths a year in the UK, mainly due to respiratory, cardiac and neurological problems (Box 14.8). Be aware it can take many hours to develop all the CVS effect.

Management

These patients require continuous ECG monitoring and early transportation to hospital. Specific therapy is directed at minimising further GI absorption and treating dysrhythmias and asthma according to ALS and

TABLE 14.1 Signs of aspirin overdose	
Dose	Effects
Mild (300–500 mg/l)	Dizziness and tinnitus Nausea, vomiting Burn mouth sensation
Moderate (500–700 mg/l)	As above plus: Hyperventilation Tachycardia, sweaty, vasodilated Gastritis Increased temp Restlessness
Severe (> 700 mg/l)	As above plus: Agitation, delirium and coma Heart failure Renal failure Pulmonary oedema

---

BOX 14.8 Signs of beta-blocker overdose

- Bradycardia, dysrhythmia and PEA arrest
- Hypotension
- Bronchospasm
- Coma and convulsions

BTS guidelines. Bolus IV injection of glucagon is also commonly given as it bypasses the receptor blockade.

Opiates

This is the commonest cause of drug-related death, typically following an accidental overdose in those who misuse drugs. Respiratory depression is the most common immediate problem which can progress to a full cardiorespiratory arrest should the hypoxia be untreated. Therapy is discussed above.

Paracetamol

This is the commonest drug to be taken as an overdose. However even a severe paracetamol overdose can have very few symptoms initially and examination is almost always normal (Box 14.9). The history is therefore very important in identifying serious overdoses in the early stages (Box 14.10).

> **BOX 14.9 Symptoms of a paracetamol overdose**
>
> ■ Nausea, vomiting
> ■ Hypoglycaemia
> ■ Later clotting abnormality as prelude to developing liver failure
> ■ Renal failure

> **BOX 14.10 Clues for serious paracetamol overdose**
>
> ■ In adult significant is >12 g or >150 mg/kg/day
> ■ Presentation >8 hours from OD
> ■ Staggered OD
> ■ Renal failure
> ■ PMH indicating a reduced threshold for liver damage – alcohol abuse; taking liver enzyme inducing drugs and reduced glutathione stores (eating disorder, HIV, cystic fibrosis)

Management

At scene there is no specific treatment for a paracetamol overdose. Provide basic ABC care, measure the BM as it can be low and transport the patient to hospital. Upon arrival therapy is dictated by the plasma level measured 4 hours after ingestion. N-acetyl cysteine (NAC) is an antidote that is extremely effective as long as it is given within 8 hours of ingestion. Patients who take 'staggered' overdose are therefore difficult to evaluate. They will require blood level on arrival and 4 hours later. If the plasma level is high or rising by over 50% NAC is given.

Antidepressant drugs

Selective serotonin reuptake inhibitors (SSRIs)

A variety of effects result from the excess serotonin following an overdose of SSRIs (Box 14.11). This becomes more likely if a combination of SSRIs is taken or they are mixed with serotonergic drugs (lithium, L-tryptophan, pentazocine, clomipramine) or MAOI.

Management

These patients require basic ABC care at scene, cannulation and treatment of any fits before transportation to hospital. This management plan will then continue as the patient recovers without any specific intervention. Occasionally intensive therapy is required to deal with a serotonin syndrome which can have marked neurological and metabolic effects.

> ### BOX 14.11 Effects due to increase in serotonin (5HT)
>
> - Nausea and vomiting
> - Fever
> - Tachycardia
> - Mydriasis
> - Lethargy, agitation, confusion, fit
> - Tremor, myoclonus, hyper-reflexia

Tricyclic antidepressants

Fortunately since the introduction of SSRIs, less people are taking overdoses of this type of antidepressants. The main problem with the drug is it affects up to five different receptors in the body. These can have a variety of effects, some of which are conflicting (Table 14.2). Consequently treatment of a specific dysrhythmia or neurological effect can lead to a marked over-correction.

TABLE 14.2 Tricyclic antidepressant drugs – site of action and affect

Receptor & mechanism	Site	Effect
Atropine-like (anti-cholinergic)	Muscarinic Central Peripheral	Anxiety, agitation – fitting Hallucinations, delirium Pyrexia Dilated pupils Dry mouth Constipation Tachyarrhythmia Urinary retention Hyperpyrexia Delayed gastric emptying
Phenothiazine-like (α-adrenergic blockade)	Central Peripheral	Sedation Vasodilatation Fall in BP
Cocaine-like (block uptake of NAdr)	Central α Peripheral α and β	Psychomotor activation Tachyarrhythmia Hypertension
Reserpine-like (catecholamine depletion)	Central Peripheral	Sedation, coma Fall in BP Decrease cardiac output Shock
Quinidine-like (membrane stabilisation)	Myocardium Conducting pathway	Decrease cardiac output Heart block (any) Increase in QTc, PR, QRS Increase in automaticity & arrhythmias

All major complications and signs of toxicity will occur within 6 hours of ingestion.

Management

It is possible to have a fatality from a tricycles overdose up to 5 days post-ingestion but this is in people who have been demonstrating toxicity all along. These patients therefore require ABC care, monitoring and cannulation at the scene. Dysrhythmias and fits should be managed using the standard protocols. There is no specific antidote but IV bicarbonate should be considered if the patient is having compromising dysrhythmias and is shocked.

TIP

A typical presentation of a tricyclic overdose is a drowsy patient with dilated pupils and a tachycardia

Volatile substance abuse

These are hydrocarbons that are inhaled and are very lipid soluble. Consequently they have a big effect on fat organs, including the brain (Box 14.12). The main problem is that the plasma levels required to get the euphoriant effect lie close to the toxic level. At this point the myocardium is very sensitive to catecholamines and hypoxia. Any shock, frights or exercise can precipitate dysrhythmias, including VF.

BOX 14.12 **Acute effect of volatile substances**

- 'High' – euphoria and inebriation to psychosis
- Dizzy, disorientated, slurred speech
- Bizarre behaviour, fitting
- Hypoxia (due to oxygen being displaced from alveoli), pneumonitis, acute eosinophilic pneumonia
- Bronchospasm, coughing
- Dysrhythmia, chest pain

Management

In a non-threatening manner remove the volatile substance from the patient and provide oxygen. Provide supportive ABC care, continuous cardiac monitoring and transport the patient to hospital.

Summary

Overdose and self harm are common life-threatening emergencies. The psychological dimension to assessment and treatment is as important as the management of physical problems. There is a high incidence of suicide in this group of patients and their problems should always be taken seriously.

A good knowledge of the issues of consent and assessment of capacity to make informed decisions is important. Judgements in this area can be difficult and seek an immediate further opinion in these circumstances.

Further reading

Clarke S, Dargan P 2002 Discharge of patients who have taken an overdose of opioids. Emerg Med J 19:250–251

Clarke S F J, Dargan P I, Jones A L 2005 Naloxone in opioid poisoning: walking the tightrope. Emerg Med J 22:612–616

Dargan P I, Wallace C I, Jones A L 2002 An evidence based flowchart to guide the management of acute salicylate (aspirin) overdose. Emerg Med J 19:206–209

Internet sources

British National Formulary– www.bnf.org/bnf/bnf/current/index.htm (5 Mar 2007)

Joint Royal Colleges Ambulance Service Liaison Committee– www.asancep. org.uk/JRCALC/ (5 Mar 2007)

Toxbase– www.spib.axl.co.uk (5 Mar 2007)

Mental illness assessment, management of depression and self harm; the Mental Health Act

Introduction

Mental health problems present in between 30% and 60% of primary care consultations.[1] One in six men and one in four women will suffer from a mental illness at some point in their lives.[2,3] GPs, for example, find that at least 30% (or 1.5 days per week) of their working week concerns mental health consultations. For depression alone, prevalence amongst the adult population in the UK varies between 17–71 per thousand for men and 25–124 per thousand for women.

Unfortunately these patient presentations in primary care are frequently complex and do not always fit easily into diagnostic categories.[4] The objectives of this chapter are listed in Box 15.1.

> **BOX 15.1 Chapter objectives**
>
> ■ The recognition of primary survey positive patients and those with complex but not immediately life-threatening presentations (primary survey negative patients)
> ■ The secondary survey, history taking and examination of the patient with signs or symptoms of mental illness
> ■ To describe mental health assessment and differential diagnoses with specific reference to depression and deliberate self harm
> ■ To discuss alternatives to admission, treatment and options for referral
> ■ To clarify definitions of mental disorder
> ■ To summarise the Mental Health Act (1983)
> ■ Assessment of valid consent and capacity

Primary survey

A mental illness may cause a patient to take an overdose or injure themselves in such a way that they develop immediately life-threatening ABCD problems. These problems are covered in Chapter 14.

An immediately life-threatening psychiatric situation is where the patient wants to kill themselves, or harm others (Box 15.2), but will not comply with treatment. Management will depend on a large number of factors – not only your assessment of the problem but also the extent and availability of local services.

Enlisting the support of family and carers is often the simplest and best way to resolve such conflicts. However if this does not work you will have to call for assistance. This may be the patient's own primary care team or the mental health team. In extreme situations where you judge that there is an immediate threat to the wellbeing of the patient, or others, you should call the police.

The Mental Health Act (MHA), in Section 63, states that the detained (or 'sectioned') patient's consent is not needed for medical treatment for mental disorder (when this is under the direction of the Responsible Medical Officer). This is detailed as being:

a. immediately necessary to save the patient's life; or
b. which (not being irreversible) is immediately necessary to prevent a serious deterioration of his condition; or
c. which (not being irreversible or hazardous) is immediately necessary to alleviate serious suffering by the patient; or
d. which (not being irreversible or hazardous) is immediately necessary and represents the minimum interference necessary to prevent the patient from behaving violently or being a danger to himself or to others.

However, the MHA does not necessarily permit the compulsory treatment of a physical disorder in a patient who is not consenting.

> **BOX 15.2 Indicators of life-threatening behavioral problems (a positive primary survey)**
>
> ■ The patient is threatening to kill or seriously harm themselves
> ■ The patient is a risk or danger to themselves or to others
> ■ The patient, through lack of appreciation of the consequences, is likely to come to harm
> ■ The patient, through lack of capacity, is vulnerable to abuse from others
> ■ The patient has become acutely confused

Secondary survey

If it is obvious that the patient is going to have to be assessed by another professional then only a brief evaluation will be required. However the following steps need to be taken to ensure the patient is suffering from a mental illness and not a physical disorder. Acute infections, intoxications, drug withdrawal syndromes, diabetes and neurological conditions are common physical conditions that may present with symptoms of mental illness/disorder. An acute confusional state may present very rapidly, especially in older patients. In the elderly this frequently can result from chest or urinary tract infections, recent life change, or progressive dementia.

Medical assessment is indicated if:

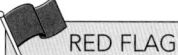

RED FLAG

Before making a psychiatric diagnosis ensure the patient is not suffering from a physical disorder

■ fever
■ history of recent fit
■ impaired or depressed level of consciousness
■ known diabetic
■ loss of awareness of surroundings
■ recent onset of confusion, disorientation and memory impairment
■ signs of head injury/recent history of head injury (2 weeks)
■ suspected chest or urinary tract infection.

Mental health assessment

While it is difficult to completely separate the mental health assessment into 'history' and exam sections, it aids understanding to use the SOAPC system. Effective mental health assessment requires a very sensitive consultation style to gain the patient's trust and showing the patient that you recognise their distress and experience. Some key principles for the mental health interview are identified in Box 15.3. Consultation skills that improve identification of emotional distress include frequent eye contact, relaxed posture, use of open questions at the beginning of the

---

> **BOX 15.3 Common signs and symptoms of mental illness**
>
> - Changes in the nature of mood (affect)
> - Disorders of perception – hallucinations and illusions
> - Disorders of thinking (cognition) – delusions, negative thinking
> - Patient's appearance and behaviour
> - Speech and communication

consultation, use of minimal verbal prompts while actively listening and avoiding giving information too early in the consultation.

Subjective – history

History taking can be difficult and at times confusing but the use of the standard template for history will help give structure and avoid omission. Elicit the main presenting complaint(s) and the onset and progress of symptoms. Is this an acute problem or more long term? Are there factors that make the symptoms better or worse? Is there a previous history of similar problems and is the patient currently undergoing treatment for these symptoms? Note the drug history, including the patient's compliance with any treatment. Is there any history of abuse of alcohol or illicit drugs? Note the past medical and psychiatric history.

Information from carers is often of great importance in the assessment. If carers are not present and you are having difficulty, you may have to trace them and discuss the issues (preferably with consent of the patient). Box 15.4 summarises the assessment of a patient with psychiatric symptoms.

> **BOX 15.4 Mental health – history**
>
> - Presenting problem
> - History of onset and progress of presenting problem
> - Previous medical history
> - Drug history/allergies/compliance with treatment
> - Past psychiatric history
> - Previous contact with services
> - Carer information

Objective information – mental state examination

Perform a brief physical exam, including noting the vital signs (especially pulse, temperature and Glasgow Coma Score). Listing the elements of a mental state examination is an excellent way to bring some structure to what can be a confusing and difficult task. These key elements are listed in Box 15.5. The assessment of social support is often of the greatest importance in deciding a management plan.

> **BOX 15.5 Elements of a mental state examination**
>
> - A – appearance
> - B – behaviour (normal, flat, manic, tremor)
> - C – cognition, concentration, memory, attention span, thought process (logical, flight, tangential)
> - D – Delusions and ideation (suicidal, homicidal), hallucinations
> - E – energy and motivation
> - Also assess risk to self and others, of deliberate self harm (DSH), impulsivity, signs of abuse of drugs or alcohol, current carer or family support, coping strategies

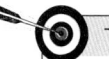

TIP

Talk to the family and get their viewpoint

This process can be difficult but allow the patient to explain the problem in their own words. Be non-judgemental. Try to help the patient focus on the issues to enable them to gain self-control. Seek clarification by the use of paraphrasing, reflection and summarising. Share your impressions. Do not be afraid to use periods of silence.

Analysis

At the end of the assessment you should be able to judge if the patient has:

- a physical disorder
- a disorder of mood (commonly depression)
- acute anxiety or panic
- acute confusion
- a psychotic disorder
- or is threat to themselves or others.

Depression

Depression is the most common mental disorder in primary care and covers a range of mental health diagnoses and problems. These are all distinguished by lowered mood and a loss or decrease of interest and pleasure in daily life and experiences. Additionally, there are disorders of thinking, problem-solving and behavioural and physiological symptoms.[5] Box 15.6 lists the diagnostic criteria for severe depression but it is often difficult to discriminate between normal mood variations, dysthymia (Box 15.7) and cyclothymic (Box 15.7) episodes and mild to moderate clinical depression.

It is not clear how effective practitioners are at preventing suicide. A number of patients who successfully commit suicide will have consulted a healthcare professional in the immediately preceding period. At least 30% see their GP in the 4 weeks prior to their deaths.[6] Improving the recognition of severe depression and its treatment has been the focus

> **BOX 15.6 Recognition and classification of severe (major) clinical depression**
>
> At least **5** of the following symptoms are **consistently** experienced by the client on a daily basis over a **2-week period**:
> - persistent sad mood
> - loss of interest or pleasure in activities that were once enjoyed
> - significant weight loss or gain without dieting, increased or reduced appetite
> - insomnia or hypersomnia
> - psychomotor agitation or retardation
> - fatigue or listlessness, loss of energy
> - feelings of worthlessness and inappropriate guilt
> - reduced ability to concentrate, make decisions or think recurrent thoughts of death or suicidal ideation

> **BOX 15.7 Differential diagnoses – mood disorders**
>
> - Clinical depression
>   - severe
>   - moderate
>   - mild
> - Bipolar disorder (manic depression)
> - Dysthymic episodes – chronic low grade depression (for at least 2 years)
> - Cyclothymia – cycling variations in mood; much less extreme than in manic depression
> - Seasonal affective disorder
> - Post-natal depression
> - Psychotic depression

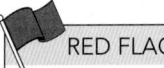

RED FLAG

Patients with mental illness have an increased risk of suicide

RED FLAG

Believe the patient when they say they will try to kill or harm themselves

of several studies and training packages for GPs but the long-term data show little sustained difference.

It is often helpful to support the patient in 'telling their story' – what a typical day is like, what makes it better or worse and listening carefully not only to 'what' they say but 'how' they express their narrative.

Each year people with depression account for two-thirds of all deaths from suicide nationally (Box 15.8). Risk assessment tools and rating scales can be very helpful, e.g. the Suicide and Self-Harm Risk Assessment Scale (see Chapter 14).

Treatment and referral

Prior to the Mental Health National Service Framework (MHNSF) the traditional management of the at-risk suicidal patient was by admission to an acute mental health unit. In non-scheduled and out-of-hours care, this may be difficult due to bed shortages, high acute in-patient bed

---

BOX 15.8 Additional risk factors for suicide

- Up to 4 weeks following discharge from services
- Recent self harm; history of violent self harm (half of those who commit suicide will have self-harmed in the past[10,11])
- Depression – paradoxically as a patient starts to recover from severe depression they regain the capacity to act
- Choice of method
- Young Asian women
- Some occupations and social groups – dentists, doctors, farmers
- Unemployed, homeless or living alone, students, divorced, separated or widowed (men)
- Relationship problems
- Chronic illness: including HIV/AIDS, cancer, diabetes, post-stroke (especially when communication centres affected), Parkinson's disease, Huntington's disease and Alzheimer's disease (where some insight remains)
- Care givers without adequate social support/finances – especially carers of those who are severely cognitively impaired
- Chronic pain

BOX 15.9 Treatment options

1. Admission to hospital:
   - severe depression, especially when suicide has been attempted or serious suicide ideation is present and the patient requires close or constant observation
2. ED and EAU Mental Health Assessment Liaison Team:
   - full psychosocial assessment (as recommended by NICE[10,11]) and referral or brief interventions offered as appropriate; may offer specific alcohol and substance misuse service
3. Home Treatment and Crisis Resolution via local mental health OOH services:
   - full psychosocial assessment and service provision for the patient with mental illness who can be supported/treated at home without admission
4. Medication:
   - this will usually be following a full mental health assessment fluoxetine or paroxetine may be prescribed for moderate to severe depression
5. Talking treatments:
   - referral to mental health team/GP – *not appropriate for people with severe depression*

---

occupancy (often in excess of 100%) and implementing MHA processes for detaining at-risk patients unwilling to agree to admission. Currently there is growth in managing these patients in the community with Crisis Resolution and Home Treatment Teams (CRHTTs) (Box 15.9). These offer intensive community-based interventions in the patient's own home (MHNSF target of 335 CRHTTs by 2005). Where such teams exist, a referral both 'in-hours' and 'out-of-hours' to the local CRHTT should be made. The CRHTT will undertake a comprehensive mental health and risk assessment. As appropriate, a treatment, support or monitoring package will be implemented.

Other alternatives to admission that may be available include acute day hospital care, psychiatric intensive care beds and assertive outreach or assertive community treatment teams. Services are, however, very variable between primary care trusts and the community practitioner will need to be familiar with the local organisation. It is therefore useful remembering that liaison nurses in emergency and MAU departments of acute general hospitals are a useful information resource for both in-patient and primary care practitioners.

Principles of effective shared and out-of-hours care

The interface between emergency care and mental health teams can be one of the most difficult to organise. This can be aided by planning. Where a patient is known, especially if they have frequent needs for emergency care, develop crisis care plans with agreed contact points. Agree out-of-hours (OOH) arrangements and ensure they are available to all relevant team members including locums.

Clarify criteria for referral and discharge between primary and secondary care; between OOH and mental health crisis teams. Develop mental health registers in primary care and joint inter-professional and multi-agency education, e.g. suicide assessment and risk management.

Consistent and regular communication with regular liaison meetings will facilitate a systematic review of shared care and complex patients. Rotations between OOH services and mental health services and regular audit will also help closer working.

Differentiating between suicide and deliberate self-harm

The MHNSF indicates that overall the rate of suicide is dropping.[7] Men are 3× more likely than women to commit suicide; women are 3–4× times more likely to present with deliberate self-harm by overdosing, cutting or other means.[8] Whilst suicide is rare, a population of 250 000 would have about 25 suicides per annum. The term deliberate self-harm (DSH) indicates that the person hurts themselves, either to signal distress, in crisis and where coping strategies are limited and to release/ manage overwhelming feelings.[9] Whilst there may be no 'intention' to kill themselves the person who is self-harming does increase the risk of death with each occasion of this behaviour. NICE identify that there are

BOX 15.10 **Relevant services and help lines**

- Bristol Crisis Line (national part-time help line)
- Community Mental Health Team
- CRHTT
- Mental Health Liaison Nurses – ED; MAU
- National Self-Harm Network
- Primary Care Gateway (Link) Workers

RED FLAG

Do not diminish the behaviour or judge it as (only) attention-seeking

150 000 attendances at A&E each year resulting from DSH – therefore being one of the top five causes of acute medical admission.[10]

So why do patients self-harm? Four main themes regarding motivation emerge from experiential and empirical research evidence. Some find this the best way of handling and expressing overwhelming feelings or of escaping numbness/unreality and confirming one's existence. It can be a method of obtaining or maintaining a sense of control. In some it is a continuation of past abusive patterns (adapted from Doy[8]). Behaviour always has a meaning – we often do not appreciate what it means for the person.

At times of crisis it is easy to disempower the person who has self-harmed by dismissing their often frustrating and repetitive behaviour as 'manipulative'. Such patients are often overwhelmed and chaotic with limited coping strategies, low self-esteem and perceptions of a lack of control and safety in their lives.

If the client is not primary survey positive undertake a psychosocial and needs assessment and a risk assessment (see Chapter 14). Recognise the distress associated with deliberate self-harm and treat the person with respect. Assume the patient has the capacity to make decisions about their care unless there is evidence to the contrary. Offer full information and seek consent to make appropriate referrals.

You may provide the patient with alternatives to self-harming including help-line contact and for pre-hospital workers to consider referral for psychotherapy. Many social care or voluntary agencies may be effective in supporting the patient with relationship, accommodation, financial, substance misuse, abuse and violence issues (Box 15.10).

Mental health and its management in community settings is complex. The key challenges include developing competence in assessment and risk assessment, in clarifying roles and services in the OOH/emergency contexts and drawing up clear and agreed guidelines and communication channels. Underpinning a number of these actions is the Mental Health Act.

The Mental Health Act

Patients who have a mental disorder requiring immediate treatment commonly consent to treatment. Only around 10% of those admitted to Mental Health Hospitals are there against their will under a 'Section' of the Mental Health Act (MHA).

In situations where a person is suffering from a 'Mental Disorder' and refuses intervention for that Mental Disorder, then the Authority for intervention may be the Mental Health Act (1983). Key to the understanding of the MHA are the definitions of *mental disorder*. The definitions are legal terms, but the diagnosis of a type of Mental Disorder is a matter for clinical judgement. Use of alcohol and other substances might sometimes cause a Mental Disorder which is within the scope of the Act, but use of these substances in itself is not within the scope of the Act.

Only a small number of professionals are involved in applying the Mental Health Act (MHA), principally Approved Social Workers (ASWs), GPs and doctors approved under Section 12 of the Act (either psychiatrists or others with experience in mental health who have been certified by the Department of Health). Each professional completing a recommendation for detention performs a detailed assessment of the patient's mental state and circumstances. If any one of them feels there is insufficient evidence to recommend detention, the person cannot be kept in hospital. [Mental health law is currently under review, the draft Mental Health Bill is currently receiving detailed scrutiny (and engendering great debate) prior to enactment in due course. The MHA (1983) therefore is the current mental health legislative guidance.]

Definitions

Mental Disorder is defined as: 'mental illness, arrested or incomplete development of mind, psychopathic disorder and any other disorder or disability of mind'.

The four sub-categories of Mental Disorder are further defined.

1 Mental illness

There is no legal definition but there are many terms and definitions, see for example the JRCALC Clinical Practice Guidelines[11] or the International Classification of Diseases, version 10.[12] Mental illness may be defined as a number of conditions typically involving impairment of an individual's normal cognitive (thinking), emotional, or behavioural functioning. It can be precipitated by biopsychosocial, biochemical, normal and traumatic life events, genetic or other factors, including infection or head injury.

The following are some of the potential characteristics of mental illness presentations:

- impairment of intellectual functions shown by a failure of memory, disorientation, difficulties in comprehension or learning capacity
- persistent alteration of mood affecting the patient's daily life

- delusional beliefs
- abnormal perceptions (hallucinations) associated with delusional beliefs and thinking patterns
- disordered thinking (cognition) which prevents the patient exercising judgement and perceiving the consequence of their actions.

2 Severe mental impairment

'A state of arrested or incomplete development of mind which includes severe impairment of intelligence and social functioning and is associated with abnormally aggressive or seriously irresponsible conduct on the part of the person concerned.'

3 Mental impairment

'A state of arrested or incomplete development of mind (not amounting to severe mental impairment) which includes significant impairment of intelligence and social functioning and is associated with abnormally aggressive or seriously irresponsible conduct on the part of the person concerned.'

4 Psychopathic disorder

'A persistent disorder or disability of mind (whether or not including significant impairment of intelligence) which results in abnormally aggressive or seriously irresponsible conduct on the part of the person concerned.'

Treatment options

In an emergency situation the police have powers of arrest under section 136 of the MHA. Under section 136 the police may remove the patient to a place of safety for detention for up to 72 hours. The patient may be detained within that time period by anyone accepting custody from the police, and a place of safety can include an NHS hospital, police station, mental health nursing home, residential home for the mentally disordered, social services residential accommodation, or any other suitable place if the occupier is willing.

It is important to note that Section 136 does *NOT* include the power to impose treatment without consent. The patient has the right to consult a solicitor in private and to have a person of their choice present.

The presence of Mental Disorder does not in itself render the individual unable to give Valid Consent. Valid Consent is always 'situation specific'. An individual who has a Mental Disorder may be able to give Valid Consent for some things, but not for others.

Fig. 15.1 Use of the Mental Health Act.

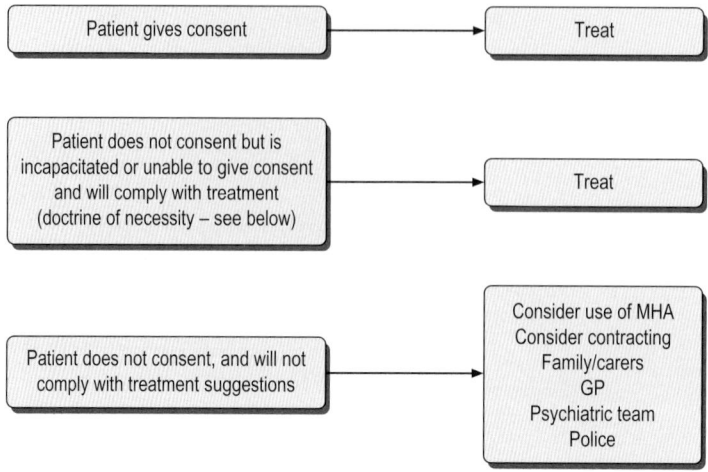

Use of the MHA is strictly defined (Fig. 15.1). 'Informal' patients are either:

- 'admitted and treated with their valid consent'

    or:

- 'incapacitated and unable to give valid consent', so:

    admitted and treated under the Common Law doctrine of:

- 'necessity'
- acting in the patient's 'best interests'
- under a 'duty of care'.

If an incapacitated patient Dissents, and the Dissent is 'persistent and purposeful' – then an Assessment should be made for compulsory Treatment under the Mental Health Act.

A ruling by the European Court of Human Rights (October 5, 2004), regarding the 'Bournewood' case may have significant impact on the use of Common Law to admit and treat Incapacitated Adults. At the time of writing the UK Government is considering their position regarding this ruling.

Most importantly, unless the patient has been detained under a relevant section of the MHA (currently section 3), if they have capacity they may legally refuse treatment, even if they are suffering from a mental disorder. Even if detained under section 3, only treatment for the mental disorder can be legally imposed in a patient with capacity. Treatment for a physical disorder which is not associated with the mental illness cannot be imposed under these circumstances.

Assessment of valid consent

An underlying principle of medical care is that consent should always be sought before any intervention is commenced. Treatment without valid consent may lead to charges of assault, or battery or worse, but there are situations where it is necessary to treat a patient without consent. There is sometimes a difficult conflict between the patient's right to determine their own treatment and the professional responsibility to act 'in the patient's best interests'. Failure to intervene and care for a patient who cannot give valid consent may lead to charges of negligence.

The Mental Capacity Act[13] gives clear guidance in this area. A good understanding of the principles of this legislation and its application to practice empowers not only the practitioner, but also the patients with whom we work.

In a large majority of cases the authority for examination and treatment is established by the patient giving their valid consent. Issues of consent in children are discussed in Chapter 5 (pages 87–89). The discussion in this section applies to adults. Valid consent comprises four components. The absence of any one component will render the consent invalid. For consent to be valid the patient should be able to:[14]

- understand relevant information about the decision to be made
- retain that information
- use the information as part of the decision-making process and understand the consequences of their decision
- communicate their decision.

We must give the patient adequate information so that they can make an informed choice. The law requires that we inform the patient of the 'broad terms of the nature of the procedure'. In the time pressured environment of emergency care it is not possible to discuss every detail of management, but we should try to ensure the patient has adequate information on which to base a decision.

We must ensure that neither we, nor anyone else, put undue pressure on the patient to comply with our wishes to intervene.

Capacity

Does the patient have 'capacity' to consent? Assessment of a patient's capacity to make a decision about their own health care is a matter of clinical judgement, guided by current professional practice and subject to the legal requirements of the Mental Capacity Act. It is the responsibility of any healthcare professional proposing treatment to determine the patient has capacity to give valid consent.

An individual is presumed to have capacity unless you have good grounds to suspect they lack capacity. If the patient appears not to have capacity to consent, then reasonable steps should be taken to help

BOX 15.11 **The capacity test**

- Is the person able to take in and retain information material to the decision, especially as to the likely consequences of having, or not having the treatment?
  or:
- Is the patient unable to weigh the information in the balance, as part of the process of arriving at the decision?

the individual understand the situation. Capacity will be affected by common trauma situations such as, shock, pain or fear.

Treatment without consent

There will be some instances where care or treatment is needed, but the patient is unable to give valid consent. At times it is obvious that you need to act without consent, for example the patient is unconscious. In other situations the decision might be less clear, for example in patients with dementia or a mental disorder. If there is time, it is advisable to ask for help and a second opinion but this is not always possible.

If an adult patient is unable to give valid consent then a healthcare professional can decide to treat the patient. We must be able to demonstrate that:

- our interventions are necessary to save life or prevent deterioration of the situation
- our interventions are in 'the patient's best interests'
- any action or treatment should be proportionate and necessary.

Even if a patient lacks capacity there is a fundamental need to ensure they are given an explanation of what is to happen.

Patients detained under the Mental Health Act can still retain capacity and that consent may still be required to provide certain forms of treatment.

Summary of principles[13]

- A person must be assumed to have capacity unless it is established that they lack capacity.
- A person should not be treated as lacking capacity unless all *practicable* steps to help them decide have been taken without success.
- A person is not to be treated as unable to make a decision merely because they make an unwise decision.
- A decision made on behalf of a person who lacks capacity must be made in their best interests.
- If a patient lacks capacity and you elect to treat the patient without their consent, plan a course of action that has least effect on the person's rights and freedom of action.

References

1 Mental Health After Care Association 1999 First national GP survey of mental health in primary care. MACA, London
2 Department of Health 1999 Modern standards and service models: mental health. NHSE, London
3 National Institute for Health and Clinical Excellence 2004 Depression: the management of depression in primary and secondary care. Available online: http://www.nice.org.uk/ (5 Mar 2007)
4 Mynors-Wallis L, Moore M, Maguire J, Hollingbery T 2002 Shared care in mental health. Oxford University Press, Oxford
5 World Health Organization 2000 WHO Guide to mental health in primary care. Royal Society of Medicine, London
6 Evans J 2002 Suicide, deliberate self-harm, and severe depressive illness. In: Elder A, Holmes J (eds) Mental health in primary care. OUP, Oxford
7 Department of Health 2002 National suicide prevention strategy for England. DoH, London
8 Doy R 2003 Women and deliberate self-harm. In: Boswell G, Poland F (eds) Women's minds, women's bodies: an interdisciplinary approach to women's health. Palgrave Macmillan, Basingstoke
9 Burstow B 1992 Radical feminist therapy: working in the context of violence. Sage, London
10 National Institute for Health and Clinical Excellence 2004 Self-harm: the short-term physical and psychological management and secondary prevention of self-harm in primary and secondary care. Available online: http://www.nice.org.uk (5 Mar 2007)
11 Joint Royal Colleges Ambulance Liaison Committee 2004 Clinical practice guidelines version 3.0. University of Warwick/ASA/JRCALC. Available online: http://www.nelh.nhs.uk/emergency (5 Mar 2007)
12 World Health Organization 1992 ICD-10 Classification of mental and behavioural disorders. WHO, Geneva
13 http://www.dca.gov.uk/menincap/legis.htm#reldocs
14 http://www2.warwick.ac.uk/fac/med/research/hsri/emergencycare/jrcalc_2006/guidelines

Further reading

BMA 1999 The Mental Health Act 1983: Guidance for general practitioners: medical examinations and medical recommendations under the Act. BMA, London
Department of Health 2001 Reference guide to consent for examination or treatment. DoH, London
Hatton C, Blackwood R 2003 Examination of the mental state. In: Lecture notes on clinical skills, 4th edn. Blackwell Science, Oxford
National Institute for Health and Clinical Excellence. The NICE website contains clinical guidelines for depression and anxiety, also for schizophrenia and self-harm– www.nice.org.uk (5 Mar 2007)

Rosie Doy, Elizabeth Jane Blowers and Emma Sutton

Assessing and managing psychosis, drug misuse and violence and aggression

Primary survey

The objectives of this chapter are listed in Box 16.1. Assess the risk of self harm or the potential of harm to others, including you. Call for urgent back up if this is the case. You may need to call the police if you think there are real and immediate risks of violence. If you judge management of the patient will require the use of the Mental Health Act, you will need to mobilise an Approved Social Worker (ASW), the patient's GP or a doctor approved under Section 12 of the Mental Health Act (1983).

BOX 16.1 **Chapter objectives**

Psychotic illness
- To discuss the recognition of psychosis in primary survey positive patients and those with non-life-threatening psychotic presentations
- To describe mental health assessment, differential diagnoses and therapeutic approaches to the person with psychotic symptoms
- To clarify referral and care pathways

Substance misuse
- To identify the tiers and responsibilities related to substance misuse service delivery
- To discuss first-line assessment and recognition of problems related to substance misuse and appropriate care pathways
- To explore psychosocial issues, co-morbidity and care strategies for primary survey negative patients who have misused drugs

Violence and aggression
- To clarify the challenge of violence and aggression in health care
- To explore reasons why violence and aggression occur
- To discuss personal and scene safety, the use of the assault cycle, de-escalation skills and post-incident staff support

Psychotic illness

This section will discuss:

- the differentiation between psychotic illness and an organic acute confusional state
- schizophrenia
- bipolar disorders (manic depression)
- post-natal psychosis.

Around 1% of the population experience at least one acute episode of schizophrenia[1] and a similar number will be affected by bipolar disorder (manic depression) at some time during their lives. Post-natal depression and psychosis is now the leading cause of all maternal deaths by suicide.

Features of psychosis and differentiation from organic confusion

In psychosis, the person typically loses the ability to distinguish between reality and thoughts due to hallucinations or delusions. These symptoms usually first appear in the late teens or early twenties (slightly later for women).

The symptoms of psychosis can be difficult to categorise. Disturbance of thought is key to the diagnosis. This thought disturbance can take

---

BOX 16.2 **Signs and symptoms of psychosis**

- *Delusions* – false, fixed beliefs that are not amenable to change despite objective and contradictory evidence to the contrary
- *Hallucinations* – disordered perception of senses including hearing voices (auditory), visual, taste (gustatory), smell (olfactory), feeling strange sensations (tactile) – these may cause the person to act on their perceptions
- *Mood (affect) disturbances*
- *Social isolation, withdrawal and apathy* – poor social and living skills, self-neglect
- *Thought (cognitive) disturbances* – the person may believe that thoughts are being inserted into or taken out of their mind; or that their thoughts are being broadcast; they may have disordered thinking and communicate bizarrely or incoherently
- Unpredictable or bizarre behaviour

---

many forms. Delusions (false beliefs) and hallucinations are common. Auditory hallucinations are common – these may take the form of voices commenting on the patient's actions or voices discussing the patient. The patient may believe that thoughts are being either inserted into or removed from their mind. Overwhelming negative feelings such as apathy, neglect and severe blunting of mood are common in severe depressive syndromes (Box 16.2).

Patients who have had a previous episode of psychotic illness are likely to be known to the specialist mental health services, though many are managed completely within primary care. It is likely that most pre-hospital and emergency care practitioners will encounter patients in crisis who have an undetected illness (the incidence of new cases of schizophrenia is 1–2 per 10 000 population per year) or those experiencing a relapse.

Exclusion of an acute organic confusion

It is not always easy to distinguish between medical/physiological disorders and mental illness presentations. Medical problems are potentially treatable and may indicate a life-threatening emergency that may be amenable to treatment (Box 16.3). History of fits, diabetes, head injury,

---

BOX 16.3 **Screening for physical causation**

Medical assessment/emergency indicated if:
- fever
- history of recent fit
- impaired or depressed level of consciousness
- known diabetic
- loss of awareness of surroundings
- recent onset of confusion, disorientation and memory impairment
- signs of head injury or recent history of head injury (2 weeks)
- suspected chest or urinary tract infection (esp. in the elderly)

TABLE 16.1 Features distinguishing organic from functional causes of psychosis		
	Organic	Functional
Age	>40 years	<40 years
Onset	Sudden	Gradual
Physical abnormalities on examination	Yes	No
Activity	Hypo-/hyper-active, tremor, ataxia	Rocking, repetitive action, posturing
Consciousness	Impaired	Awake and alert
Orientation	No	Yes
Lucid thoughts	Some	Infrequent
Hallucinations	Visual	Auditory
Memory impairment	Recent memory	Remote memory

recent febrile illness or acute confusion should be excluded (a full list is given in Chapter 15). Check the temperature, level of consciousness, orientation and speed of onset as these can help distinguish between and physical or psychiatric cause (Table 16.1).

Psychiatric assessment

The objectives are to obtain an accurate history of the presenting problem, assess the patient's mental state and personality, and to identify possible causes/triggers to the current situation. In addition to the usual approach to history taking and past medical/psychiatric history of the patient, it is useful to assess the patient's expectations/wishes and their appropriateness. The patient's mental state should then be assessed; this may involve the use of the Mental State or Mini Mental State Examinations (see, for example, the Oxford Handbook of Psychiatry[2]). Another approach to mental state examination is given in Box 16.4.

The patient's presentation may be complicated by emotional arousal (e.g. anger), the misuse of alcohol and co-morbidity. An example of the latter is 'self-medication' with cannabis by patients experiencing the symptoms of schizophrenia. In the UK 9–35% of people with schizophrenia misuse alcohol or drugs.

BOX 16.4 The ABCDE model – initial psychiatric assessment

- **A** Appearance – neglected, dishevelled, inappropriate dress for weather/environment?
- **B** Behaviour – disinhibited, impulsive, bizarre, aggressive, unpredictable, withdrawn?
- **C** Communication – incoherent, rapid and disconnected, confused, limited/uncommunicative?
- **D** Ideation – beliefs, delusions, preoccupied, perception, hallucinations, thought processes?
- **E** Emotion – excitable, euphoric, suspicious, sad, flat, depressed, inappropriate to situation, rapidly changing (labile)?

Analysis

The categorisation of severe mental illness is not easy. You do not have to make a definite diagnosis – indeed it may be inadvisable to 'label' a patient in the first contact emergency situation. However it is important to have some appreciation of the main categories. These are summarised in Box 16.5.

BOX 16.5 Differential diagnoses of psychotic disorder – specific mental disorders

- Acute or transient psychotic disorder – usually associated with acute stress and resolves in 2–3 weeks
- Bipolar disorder (also called manic depression) – cyclic disorder characterised by repeated episodes of elevated mood (mania) and depression
- Persistent delusional disorder – characterised by a single delusion or set of related delusions; there are no hallucinations nor disturbances in mood, speech or behaviour
- Post-natal depression and psychosis
- Psychoactive substance abuse
- Schizophrenia
- Severe clinical depression with psychotic features

Specific types of illness

Schizophrenia

The main symptoms are of thought disorder. Belief that thoughts are being inserted or removed or transferred to the patient are common. Auditory hallucinations such as a commentary of patient's actions or a voice anticipating or repeating the patient's thoughts are often described. Delusions are common. The patient is often isolated and may exhibit apathy and blunting of mood.

TIP

Physical examination may also be necessary; schizophrenia is associated with a high mortality, with death on average 10 years earlier than the general population. Cardiovascular disease and/or diabetes are responsible for many of these excess deaths[1,4]

Develop rapport and therapeutic relationship taking account of language and culture of the patient. Involve patients and carers/advocates in care decisions. Look for a previously documented crisis care plan and check concordance with and previous response to any treatment/medication package. Assess alcohol and substance use or misuse.

In an acute episode of psychosis, especially the first experience, the person may be absolutely terrified and confused. There may be suicidal ideas (about 10% of patients with schizophrenia will commit suicide within 5 years of the onset of their illness; about 30% of people with schizophrenia attempt suicide at least once). They may 'hear' voices demanding that they harm themselves.[3] Those most at risk are male patients, the unemployed, socially isolated or recently discharged from hospital.

Bipolar disorder

Bipolar disorder is defined by NICE[5] as: 'an episodic, potentially life-long, disabling disorder (with) diagnostic features including periods of mania and depression characterised by periods of abnormally elevated mood or irritability, which may alternate with periods of depressed mood. These episodes are distressing and often interfere with occupational or educational functioning, social activities and relationships.'

The evidence shows that there is often a considerable delay between the onset of the disorder and first contact with services.

Most people experience some changes in mood, but a patient with mania (Box 16.6) has a persistently high and euphoric mood, which is out of keeping with their circumstances and the environment. A key feature of management is to provide a calm, structured environment with avoidance of over-stimulation balanced with space for walking to use up excess

---

BOX 16.6 Signs and symptoms of mania

- Bizarre or inappropriate behaviour
- Decreased sleep which may lead to exhaustion
- Delusions and hallucinations
- Elevated mood
- Enhanced libido, flirtatiousness, sexual disinhibition and promiscuity
- Flight of ideas – racing thoughts
- Grandiose ideas and inflated self-esteem
- Impaired concentration, distractibility
- Impaired judgement and decision making
- Impulsive behaviour and recklessness, disregard for danger; spending sprees
- Increased energy and activity levels
- Increased pain threshold
- Irritability, truculence and aggression
- Labile moods – quickly changing, e.g. from elation to anger
- Poor insight
- Pressure of speech which may be difficult to understand

energy. Hospital admission is therefore often necessary. In contrast, hypomania (i.e. when the symptoms are not extreme enough to significantly impair work/relationships) can be managed within primary care.

Be aware that many medications may induce the symptoms of mania including antidepressants, other psychotropic medication, anti-parkinsonian medication, cardiovascular and respiratory drugs, anti-TB medications, steroids and drugs of misuse.

Post-natal depression and psychosis

Following childbirth, around 70% of women experience 'baby blues'; this usually occurs 3–5 days after the birth and resolves quickly. However, about 10% experience post-natal depression which exhibits the same symptoms as a severe (major) depression.[6] Secondary survey would be supported by use of the Edinburgh Post-natal Depression Scale.[7]

A small percentage of new mothers (0.1%) develop puerperal psychosis (Box 16.7) – this normally develops within 3 weeks of the birth.

BOX 16.7 **Signs and symptoms of post-natal psychosis**

- Delusions and hallucinations (as indicated above)
- Feelings of guilt
- Low mood which may alternate with elation and euphoria
- Sleep disturbances
- Appetite problems
- Confusion
- Ambivalence towards the baby

This is a serious illness and may require prompt specialist intervention and the admission of the mother and baby. 'Why Mothers Die' – The Confidential Enquiry into Maternal Deaths[8] indicates clearly that 50% of the women who commit suicide (Box 16.8) have a previous history of serious mental illness, 25% related to their last childbirth. This is in fact the leading cause of maternal death. Four times as many suicides occurred following delivery than in pregnancy itself and many women with puerperal psychosis who kill themselves do so later than 6 weeks following delivery.

Appropriate in-patient services may be difficult to access depending on locality since there is a national shortfall in the number of 'mother and baby' beds available.

Responding to a person in crisis

Whatever the category of psychotic diagnosis, the development of a therapeutic relationship and effective active listening skills are key components in helping the distressed patient in the crisis situation (Box 16.9). The client needs to feel accepted and understood by a practitioner who is trustworthy, interested, helpful and understanding. Such an approach will help

BOX 16.8 Summary of findings related to women who commit suicide

- 87% were white
- 83% were over the age of 25 years
- 46% were over the age of 30 years
- 55% had previous children
- 54% were seriously ill, either suffering from a postpartum psychosis or a very severe depressive illness
- 50% had a previous history of serious illness, of whom half had been admitted to a psychiatric unit
- 50% were in contact with psychiatric services during their index maternity, 75% of whom were receiving some form of treatment
- Only one woman with significant post-partum mental illness had been admitted to a specialist mother and baby unit
- 65% of the suicides died violently, half from hanging or jumping from a height, clearly reflecting the profound disturbance of their mental state and intention to die
- Only 35% died from an overdose of prescribed medication
  These illnesses were therefore neither hidden nor undetected.

(From: Why Mothers Die[8])

to prevent violence and aggression and facilitate assessment and appropriate referral of the patient.

Services available

In the past, the first occurrence of an acute crisis or a relapse episode of psychosis led to admission to an acute inpatient bed. More recently such crises are tending to be managed in the community (Box 16.10). Crisis resolution and home treatment teams (CRHTTs) are designed to provide out-of-hours care for acutely ill patients with psychosis via intensive community home-based support and treatment, thereby avoiding the additional trauma and stigma of a hospital admission. Under the guidance of specialist mental health services rapid tranquillisation may be offered to enhance effective and early intervention and management of the patient.

In summary, effective recognition of psychotic presentations, detailed assessment including risk identification and enhanced awareness of available services will support the urgent/unscheduled care practitioner in managing the person experiencing a psychotic crisis. The assessment and crisis management approaches suggested here are supported by current clinical guidelines and NSFs and form the general principles for effective intervention for a mental health client in distress.

In the emergency care context it is acknowledged that there will frequently be time pressures, as well as lack of confidence impacting on the

---

BOX 16.9 Responding to a person in crisis

- Accept the experienced reality but do not confirm or argue with the patient's beliefs
- Acknowledge the person's feelings, e.g. anger, fear – give the patient time and space to calm down, and do not take it personally
- Avoid labels, e.g. schizophrenic, alcoholic
- Do not ask too many questions
- Do not escalate the situation
- Do not patronise
- Encourage concordance with medication
- Encourage personal control where possible
- Explain **everything**
- Gain consent before talking to the family/carers
- Help in the 'here and now' – aim is not to cure the patient but to manage the current crisis
- Listen to the person's concerns
- Look and listen for clues and incongruence in communication (mismatch between body language and what is said)
- Maintain detailed documentation
- Maintain personal and scene safety
- Make appropriate eye contact
- Plan and agree clear goals
- Reassure the patient and their family/carers
- Risk assessment and management
- Set and state clear boundaries if the person is demanding, disinhibited, etc.
- Use local referral pathways and liaise with appropriate specialist services
- Use the patient's name
- Very careful reality testing **may** be helpful, i.e. offering alternative explanations

---

BOX 16.10 Services available (these will vary according to locality)

- Acute Admission Units (however there is a national shortage of 'mother and baby' beds)
- Acute Day Hospitals
- Approved Social Worker
- Assertive Outreach/Assertive Community Teams (AOT/ACT)
- Community Mental Health Teams (CMHT)
- Crisis Resolution and Home Treatment Teams (CRHTT)
- Duty Psychiatrist
- Early Interventions Teams (EIT)
- Mental Health Link (Primary Care Gateway) Workers
- Police
- Primary Care Teams
- Self-help Groups

practitioner and team's ability to fully implement the suggested guidelines and strategies. It is therefore useful for the urgent care worker to establish and develop working relationships with liaison mental health practitioners (in A&E or emergency assessment centres), mental health crisis resolution teams, and mental health link workers (in primary care), so that urgent referrals and joint assessment protocols can be developed.

Substance misuse

Following publication of the national drug strategy, 'Tackling drugs to build a better Britain'[9] there has been increased focus on the provision of drug treatment services that will work effectively with other health, social care and criminal justice service providers in order to provide seamless treatment and care to substance misusers. As part of that strategy 'Models of Care'[10] provides the framework that is intended to achieve equity, parity and consistency in the provision of substance misuse treatment and care in the UK. Treatment tiers and services are identified that are inclusive of all healthcare settings, providing guidance on the levels of intervention, assessment and expectations of those working within a given tier. This systematic approach to service structure is also designed to enable clearer recognition and access to the appropriate tier of service following identified need (Table 16.2).

Emergency care settings are acknowledged as being a significant Tier 1 service due to the prevalence of overt or covert substance-related

TABLE 16.2 Structure of service provision for substance misusers

Tier	Service provision
Tier 1	Non-substance misuse specific services (to include primary care providers; emergency care settings; general medical inpatient settings; general psychiatric care providers)
Tier 2	Open access substance misuse services (may include NHS and independent sector; health/social care or self-referrals accepted; offering advice, brief interventions, support and counselling, low-threshold prescribing)
Tier 3	Structured community-based substance misuse service (offering structured treatment programmes including substitute prescribing programmes, detoxification, day programmes and therapies)
Tier 4	(a) Residential substance misuse specific services (offering prescribing and rehabilitation) (b) Highly specialist non-substance misuse specific services

presentations within urgent/unscheduled care. In addition it is the emergency and primary non-specialist services that commonly offer a starting point for people wishing to engage in a treatment programme. As such the necessity and value of appropriate assessment and early identification by practitioners within this field is apparent.

Emergency medical intervention may be integral to the care and recovery of a presenting substance misuser, however this chapter concentrates on the process of assessment and identification of need that form the basis of engaging with the substance misusing client.

The nature of substance misuse

Individual perceptions and experience of substance misuse will be diverse and are influenced by personal experience and beliefs, social norms, and cultural context. Diagnosis of misuse therefore has to accommodate and recognise the relevance of both objective and subjective characteristics identified within an assessment process (Box 16.11).

Discussion of substance misuse tends to emphasise cases where individuals are misusing illicit substances, however the principles and approaches described within Government strategy and this chapter would also apply to those misusing alcohol or any non-prescribed psychoactive substance.

Clinical criteria are available to aid recognition of substance misuse as a health problem, but additionally a number of more holistic and person-centred perspectives are appropriate. Substance misuse may

---

BOX 16.11 Key diagnostic criteria (not all of which may be present)

- *Compulsion and cravings.* The person describes a subjective awareness of the need or desire to take the substance. This is often strongest during attempts to reduce or stop
- *Salience.* The substance becomes an increasingly significant part of the person's life, often involving increasing frequency and quantity of substance used. Priority may be given to drug- seeking or drug-related behaviours relative to other previously valued activities
- *Neuroadaptation.* Physical symptoms of dependency may develop including tolerance and withdrawal
- *Use to avoid withdrawal.* A pattern of perpetuated or continual use may present due to either physical or psychological 'withdrawal'. This may include the absence of physical dependency whereby the person has a belief system that without the substance they will be unable to function or cope
- *Continued use despite negative effects.* This may occur even where the potential damage is quite clear to the individual
- *Reinstatement.* A rapid or repetitive return to use can be noted after a period of abstinence

refer to addiction, where physical dependence is implied, but may also include terms such as abuse, dependency or problematic usage. This varying language can cause confusion in both practitioners and individuals misusing substances, leading to potential difficulties in deciding **when** and indeed **if** the person is engaging in potentially harmful usage.

If an individual identifies their current use of a substance as causing difficulties in any aspect of wellbeing then it is helpful to accept these concerns as valid and their use should therefore be considered to be problematic. In assessing the presence of substance misuse, a number of themes or criteria are commonly considered and are reflected within both ICD[11] and DSM[12] criteria.

Assessing substance misuse

Within 'Models of Care',[10] guidelines are offered to inform how practitioners working in all tiers of service provision assess. Three levels of assessment are identified including screening and referral; triage substance misuse assessment; and comprehensive assessment.

Tier 1 services including emergency departments and unscheduled care settings are expected to demonstrate consideration of a number of themes as part of a level 1 'screening and referral' assessment (Box 16.12). It is expected that all practitioners working within this tier of service are competent in this area.

It is essential that in undertaking an assessment of substance misuse, respect and regard for the client is demonstrated. Substance misusers often have experienced a number of traumatic life events leading to their use of substances. The reasons why a person may use are complex and multifaceted[13] and as such moral judgements and assumptions are unhelpful to both the client and practitioner. Whilst practitioners in urgent and unscheduled care environments may not have the time or opportunity to explore why someone has developed a problem, they can usefully accept that whatever the reason, it is valid. A non-judgemental, open and conversational approach to assessment is advocated.

Brief interventions

Individuals presenting with 'early' problems can be usefully targeted and brief interventions offered to minimise future significant misuse and maximise long-term positive outcomes.[14] This approach has proved especially beneficial where a person does not present with overt dependence and is particularly relevant to emergency and primary care practitioners. Brief intervention (Box 16.13) is extremely effective and may take as little as 15 minutes to complete.

BOX 16.12 Tier 1 level 1: screening and referral assessment

Content of assessment
■ Identification of substance misuse problem
  – Is the person currently using a psychoactive substance?
  – If so, what substance(s), how much, by which method, how often, for how long?
  – Is usage stable, increasing?
  – Is it a problem?
  – How does the person perceive their use, are they motivated to change?
■ Identification of related or co-existing problems
  – Consider the physical, social and psychological impact of substance misuse including medical and psychiatric complications
  – Does the person present with co-morbidity? Do they have other health problems unrelated to their substance misuse?
■ Identification of risks
  – What kind of risk may the person face from the substance and mode of usage, from their own behaviours or physical/mental state, from the social/physical environment they are in?
  – What types of risk may the person present to themselves (suicide/self-harm), to others including the practitioner, to the physical environment?
■ Assessment of urgency of referral
  – The culmination of previous content gathered. Commonly informed by aspects of risk. Where a risk is identified it may be helpful to consider:
    – imminence; how soon might the risk event occur?
    – severity; how bad will it be if it happens?
    – likelihood; how likely do I think it is to happen?
    – This can be helpful in deciding the urgency of action needed

Outcome of assessment
■ Identification of an appropriate service for referral
  – Will be informed by content of assessment, and should consider the person's needs, wishes and motivation
  – A non-dependent client may benefit from immediate 'brief intervention' (see below)
  – A low risk client with relatively uncomplicated presentation and motivation may be advised of or referred to Tier 2 services
  – Complex, vulnerable or high-risk presentations where significant need and/or prescribing/detoxification are indicated might be referred directly to Tier 3 services

BOX 16.13 The components of brief intervention – FLAGS

■ F – Feedback on risk or health implications due to drug use
■ L – Listen to the patient's concerns
■ A – Advise patient about the consequences of continued drug use
■ G – Goals of treatment should be defined, e.g. to reduce or cease drug consumption
■ S – Strategies for treatment should be discussed, e.g. limit setting on use, recognising triggers to use, and accessing support. A follow-up appointment may be made

Violence and aggression

Healthcare practitioners are at risk from patients, relatives and the public generally; additionally patients also present risks to each other.[15] Ambulance trust staff are reporting an increase in violence and aggression cases and 43% of the incidents reported in acute trusts are within Accident and Emergency departments.[16] The prevention and management of these episodes is a significant challenge for the providers of primary and emergency health care. Overall within NHS organisations there are 11 incidents per 1000 staff monthly but the rate is 2.5× higher in mental health and learning disabilities trusts.

By the very nature of emergency care, individuals who come into contact with services are likely to be experiencing some form of distress. Physical and mental illness (which may include substance misuse and patients suffering from psychosis) can lead to changes in perception, which may increase misinterpretations of the intentions and actions of healthcare staff. Anxiety heightens an individual's senses. Potential cultural difficulties with non-verbal communication misunderstandings and misinterpretation as well as language may also trigger distress and frustration[17,18] (Box 16.14).

Anger is not the only prerequisite of violence and aggression. Angry people are not always violent, but a link between this powerful emotion and associated potentially dangerous behaviour is accepted. Factors which may exacerbate a person's anger are summarised in Box 16.15.

Personal and scene safety

Good risk assessment skills (Boxes 16.16 and 16.17) are necessary in the urgent/unscheduled care arena. Personal and professional safety

---

BOX 16.14 Reasons why violence and aggression occur

- Factors internal to a patient:
  - physiological arousal
  - misperception, e.g. of sounds, actions
  - psychological aspects, e.g. feelings of loss of control, anxiety, fear, acute distress
  - acute sensory deficits – hearing or sight loss leading to breakdown in communication
  - unrealistic expectations
- Staff attitudes, lack of understanding of patient expectations
- Organisational factors
- Situational and environmental factors
- Actions of others, e.g. family

(Adapted from NICE, 2005[17])

BOX 16.15 Factors which make people angry

- Lack of respect
- Not being listened to
- Loss of control
- Sense of injustice
- Discrimination
- Lack of competence in others

BOX 16.16 Summary of patient and environmental risks

- Confusion
- Alcohol or drugs
- History of violence
- Hallucinations and delusions (explored below)
- Longer than normal/expected response time
- Forced entry to gain access to patient
- Crowds – especially at clubs, pubs or concealed spaces with restricted access
- Lone workers without back-up
- Radio black spots
- Domestic violence
- Presence of others perceived as a threat (including, for example, police or security staff)

BOX 16.17 Tips for enhancing personal safety

- Good communication systems with agreed codes
- Alarm systems
- Radio provision
- Information links with police re locations
- Flagging systems
- Good quality patient information including realistic response times
- Lone workers without back up should not attend pub fights or domestic violence situations or locations with known access substance misuse or crowd difficulties

---

(Adapted from DoH 2002[19])

---

of practitioners may be largely attributed to good habits and systems. It is the good safety behaviour which is carried out *all the time* which can make the difference in potentially life-threatening situations, rather than *additional precautions taken in particular circumstances.*

The assault cycle

The assault cycle (Box 16.18) is a theoretical model which offers general advice rather than specific predictions. The *trigger phase* is a time

> **BOX 16.18 The assault cycle**
>
> **Trigger phase**
> Behaviour moves away from baseline, e.g. agitation, poor concentration, raised voice
> - *Interventions*: identify potential risks; early use of de-escalation techniques may include distraction
>
> **Escalation phase**
> Behaviour escalates
> - *Interventions*: continued use of de-escalation techniques
>
> **Crisis phase**
> Patient and staff member are both aroused and assault is imminent or occurring
> - *Interventions*: reasoning is no longer possible; manage own physiological and physical responses with an emphasis on safety of all involved – escape, use of barriers, alarms/shouting to summon help
>
> **Recovery phase**
> Patient is calming and returning to baseline
> - *Interventions*: most intervention errors occur at this stage – be aware of the potential for 'flare up'; do not attempt an exploration of the incident at this stage
>
> **Post crisis phase**
> The patient is low in mood, remorseful, guilty, ashamed, despairing
> - *Interventions*: explore the reasons for the incident; reject the behaviour not the person; ensure all others involved receive support

TIP

Helpful actions: escape (note your escape routes carefully); protect self by use of barriers; engage the support of others

at which distraction may be important. It also offers an opportunity to assess and prepare for any potential risks. *Escalation* is the phase which may lead directly to assault. These phases offer opportunities for skilled de-escalation of a situation. Within the *crisis phase* a potential assailant experiences physical and psychological arousal. Control over aggressive impulses and the ability for rational thought decreases and this may lead to assault. The practitioner will also experience physical and psychological responses that may influence their control and effectiveness. At this stage self-management with a focus on safety issues related to the client, self and others is important.

After crisis comes the *post-crisis phase* – this is where most intervention errors occur. It is vital to acknowledge the potential for events to 'flare up' as significant time is required for individuals to calm both psychologically and physiologically (often cited as at least 90 minutes). In the final *recovery phase* an assailant may be mentally and physically exhausted and is commonly remorseful, ashamed, distraught and despairing. At this stage individuals may be responsive to interventions designed to relieve guilt which reject the assaultative behaviour but not the individual as a person, understand the incident and identify strategies to prevent a recurrence. It is vital that full attention is also given to the needs of the victim.

The assault cycle makes a series of assumptions. These are that violence is often used when someone feels powerless in relation to the professional or the system. Intervention is possible at all times except the crisis phase, when physical safety is paramount. The client and the worker experience high levels of physical or psychological arousal during episodes of aggressive behaviour, and this will affect how they both behave; the practitioner should be able to access appropriate training to develop techniques to overcome this.

De-escalation

De-escalation involves the use of techniques to calm down a threatening situation and should be applied early prior to any other interventions being used (Box 16.19).

De-escalation involves self-awareness of the messages that the worker is conveying through their verbal and non-verbal communication (Box 16.20). In effective de-escalation a person shows concern and attentiveness through non-verbal and verbal responses – listening carefully, acknowledging any concerns or frustrations, and not being patronising or minimising the patient's experience. The worker's non-verbal communication is non-threatening and not provocative.

BOX 16.19 Advice to de-escalate the situation

- One person should take control and steps must be taken to manage the environment
- Where weapons are involved a staff member should ask for the weapon to be placed in a neutral location rather than handed over
- Other people may be removed from the area by moving towards a safe place and avoiding being trapped in a corner
- The aggressor may be taken to a quieter but safe area where help is at hand
- Creating space
- Enlisting support from others
- Identify potential risks from others

(Adapted from NICE 2005[20])

BOX 16.20 Key de-escalation principles

- Attend to non-verbal cues including eye contact
- Allow greater body space than normal
- Adopt a non-threatening but safe posture
- Appear calm, self-controlled and confident
- Do not appear dismissive or over-bearing
- Explain intentions giving clear, brief, assertive instructions

---

BOX 16.21 De-escalation techniques

Environmental
- One staff member to take control
- Move to a safe area
- Minimise other distractions such as noise
- Move others
- Create space
- Ensure support is close at hand
- Ask for weapons to be put down
- Consider any sensory impairments
- Attend to the cultural context

Verbal
- Minimise risks of misinterpretation
- Show concern
- Explain intentions
- Offer and negotiate realistic options
- Avoid threats
- Establish rapport and emphasise co-operation
- Give clear, brief assertive instructions
- Ask open questions
- Listen carefully to concerns – do not minimise these or be patronising

Non-verbal
- Minimise risk for misinterpretation
- Show concern
- Non-threatening posture
- Allow personal space
- Manage eye contact

(Adapted from NICE 2005[20])

The worker who has taken control asks for facts about the problem and encourages reasoning by asking open questions and inquiring about the reason for the anger. Threats are avoided. This works to establish rapport and emphasises co-operation – offering and negotiating realistic options. Expressions of anger need to be treated with appropriate measured and reasonable responses. In a crisis situation staff are responsible for taking steps to avoid provocation (Box 16.21). It is unrealistic to expect a person exhibiting disturbed/violent behaviour to simply calm down.

Post-incident support

Individuals experience emotional, cognitive and physiological reactions during the first six weeks after an assault. A single episode of violence or aggression may have a profound impact or the effects may be the result of cumulative abuse. Feelings experienced after an assault include

BOX 16.22 **Stages of CISD**

- The introduction of team and establishing ground rules
- Establishing the facts of the incident
- Exploring the thoughts, decisions and impressions of those involved
- Exploring emotional reactions
- Normalisation of post-trauma reactions, offering anticipatory guidance and advice on helpful coping
- Exploring future planning and coping including mobilisation of support
- Disengagement

(Adapted from Dyregrov 1989[21])

disbelief, helplessness and frustration, accompanied by resentment and resignation. In most cases these symptoms are resolved after the first six months. It is in this initial most vulnerable period of time when support needs to be available. It is not only the person who is assaulted that suffers; witnesses need support.

Psychological debriefing (also referred to as Critical Incident Stress Debriefing – CISD) was originally developed for use by groups of emergency workers post-incident. This is a structured, supportive approach led by a trained facilitator (Box 16.22).

There is disagreement as to the effectiveness of this approach, with some suggestion that it may actually be harmful. Individuals have varied coping strategies and it should be made very clear to those who have been involved in incidents that a range of different support is available and that attendance at debriefing is not the only option nor is it compulsory.

In summary, the effective recognition, prevention and management of violence and aggression is of central importance to emergency care staff. This is a complex area encompassing a wide range of reasons why aggression and violence occurs. Recognition and an understanding of the role that staff, patients and environmental factors play in ameliorating the outcomes in potentially explosive situations is central to the provision of high quality care. Individuals and groups of staff have a vital role to play in maintaining personal and scene safety. This will be promoted by the employment of good safety behaviour all the time, with additional precautions as indicated.

References

1 Prodigy 2004 Schizophrenia guideline. Available online: http://www.prodigy.nhs.uk/guidance.asp?gt=Schizophrenia (5 Mar 2007)
2 Semple D, Smyth R, Burns J, Darjee R, McIntosh A 2005 Oxford handbook of psychiatry. Oxford University Press, Oxford
3 Andrews G, Jenkins R 1999 Management of mental disorders, vol 2 (UK edition). World Health Organization, London

4   National Institute for Health and Clinical Excellence 2002 Schizophrenia: core interventions in the treatment and management of schizophrenia in primary and secondary care. NICE, London. Available online: http://www.nice.org.uk/pdf/CG1NICEguideline.pdf (5 Mar 2007)

5   National Institute for Health and Clinical Excellence 2004 Bipolar disorder clinical guidelines. NICE, London. Available online: http://www.nice.org.uk/guidance/cg38/niceguidance/pdf/English (5 Mar 2007)

6   Doy R, Burroughs D, Scott J 2005 ABC of community emergency care. Issues in Mental Health – consent, the law and depression – management in emergency settings. Emerg Med J 22:279–285

7   Cox J, Holden J, Sagovsky R 1987 Detection of post-natal depression: development of the 10-item Edinburgh Post-natal Depression Scale. Br J Psychiatry 150:782–876

8   RCOG 2002 Why Mothers Die 2000–2002. Report on confidential enquiries into maternal deaths in the United Kingdom. Available online: http://www.cemach.org.uk/publications/WMD2000_2002/content.htm (5 Mar 2007)

9   UKADU 1998 Tackling drugs to build a better Britain: the Government's 10-year strategy for tackling drug misuse. Department of Health, London

10 DoH 2002 Models of care for substance misuse treatment. Department of Health, London

11 WHO 1992 International classification of diseases (ICD 10) – Classification of mental and behavioural disorders. World Health Organization, Geneva

12 American Psychiatric Association 1994 Diagnostic and Statistical Manual of Diseases (DSM-IV). APA, Washington, DC

13 Peterson T 2002 Exploring substance misuse and dependence: explanations, theories and models. In: Peterson T, McBride A (eds) Working with substance misusers, a guide to theory and practice. Routledge, London

14 Hulse G, White J, Conigrave K 2002 Identifying treatment options. In: Hulse G, White J, Cape G (eds) Management of alcohol and drug problems. Oxford University Press, Oxford

15 Chambers N 1998 'We have to put up with it – don't we?' The experience of being the registered nurse on duty, managing a violent incident involving an elderly patient; a phenomethodological study. J Advanced Nursing 27:429–436

16 NAO 2003 A safer place to work: protecting NHS and ambulance trust staff. National Audit Office, London

17 National Institute for Health and Clinical Excellence 2005 The short-term management of disturbed/violent behavior in in-patient psychiatric settings and emergency departments. Clinical Guideline 25. NICE, London

18 Paterson B, Leadbetter D, McComish A 1997 De-escalation in the management of aggression and violence. Nursing Times 93(36):58–61

19 Department of Health 2002 Zero tolerance zone fact sheets. DoH, London. Available online: www.nhs.uk/zerotolerance/intr.htm (15 May 2005)

20 National Institute for Health and Clinical Excellence 2005 The short-term management of disturbed/violent behaviour in in-patient psychiatric settings and emergency departments. Clinical Guideline 25. NICE, London

21 Dyregrov A 1989 Caring for helpers in disaster situations – psychological debriefing. Disaster Management 2:25–30

Further reading

Joint Royal Colleges Ambulance Liaison Committee, 2004: Clinical Practice Guidelines version 3.0, University of Warwick/JRCALC. Available online: http://www.library.nhs.uk/emergency/ (5 Mar 2007)

Mynors-Wallis L, Moore M, Maguire J, et al 2002 Shared care in mental health. Oxford University Press, Oxford

Simon C, Everitt H, Birtwhistle J, Stevenson B 2002 Oxford handbook of general practice. Oxford University Press, Oxford

Wright S, Gray R K, Parkes J, Gournay K 2002 The recognition, prevention and therapeutic management of violence in acute in-patient psychiatry: a literature review and evidence-based recommendations for good practice. Available online: http://www.ukcc.org.uk/aDisplayDocument. aspx?DocumentID=665 (5 Mar 2007)

Index

Note: Page numbers in bold refer to **boxes** and tables and page numbers in *italics* refer to figures.